# I'd Rather Fly a Chopper

AN IAF
HELICOPTER PILOT
REMEMBERS

# I'd Rather Fly a Chopper

RAJESH ISSER

HarperCollins *Publishers* India

First published in India by HarperCollins *Publishers* 2022
4th Floor, Tower A, Building No. 10, Phase II, DLF Cyber City,
Gurugram Haryana – 122002, India
www.harpercollins.co.in

2 4 6 8 10 9 7 5 3 1



P-ISBN: 978-93-5489-254-7
E-ISBN: 978-93-5489-545-6



Typeset in 11.5/15.2 Adobe Garamond Pro at
Manipal Technologies Limited, Manipal

Printed and bound at
Thomson Press (India) Ltd

HarperCollinsIn

MIX
Paper
FSC
FSC® C010615

This book is produced from independently certified FSC® paper
to ensure responsible forest management.

*To Godavari and Vagmi.*
*And the many generations of storytellers and listeners*

# CONTENTS


Chopper–Chopper Everywhere 1

## STRANGER THAN FICTION

Strange Encounters 11

Aisa Bhi Hota Hai 37

## ACTION CHRONICLES

A Glance at Chopper Operations 65

Videshi Melee (Mela!) 105

## TOUCHING ALL CORNERS

Purabi Prakash 133

Uttari Utkrishti 155

Adbhut Andaman and Nicobar 185

Dakshin Drishtikone 192

Madhyam Mela 208

*Epilogue* 223

*About the Author* 227

# CHOPPER–CHOPPER EVERYWHERE

UBIQUITY, OR THE ability to be present anywhere, is an apt description for a helicopter, colloquially known as a 'chopper' in the Indian military. Most people are amazed that it can fly at all—but it does and like none other. The following stories and anecdotes bring out its uniqueness as a machine and also the many misfortunes awaiting a pilot who is not serious or focused on flying it!

While humour is in the mind of the beholder, these tales, like the rest of the book, bring out the funny part behind a serious job! They bring out the fun of being a chopper pilot while undertaking risky work. The aerodynamics of helicopter-flying and the accidents waiting to happen are difficult subjects even for experienced pilots. However, these stories break them down into simple and understandable 'stuff' for all readers.

**Why These Stories?**

I have been a helicopter pilot in the Indian Air Force (IAF) since January 1983. The first chopper I flew was a French Alouette III

(Chetak) at the Helicopter Training School (HTS), Hyderabad. At the end of basic training at the Air Force Academy, Hyderabad, I had fought my way to choose helicopter-flying over the more sought-after fighter-plane-flying despite scoring high in overall merit in the course. At that time, my motivation was to join the future of combat, namely, attack helicopters. It came from reading about the West (NATO) versus Soviet (Warsaw)-projected conflicts, which were so popular at that point of time.

Ironically, despite a reasonable professional record and preference expressed every year, I did not get posted to an attack-helicopter squadron. So, do I regret my choice to swim against the tide at the beginning of my career? Never! I have had the privilege and God-sent opportunity to serve and interact with citizens of India in virtually every state of this nation in very special ways. I have had opportunities to experience combat multiple times, and a lifelong window to do my bit towards nation-building. All because of a ubiquitous and versatile aviation marvel—a helicopter, or chopper.

The chopper is so versatile that it is omnipresent in all crises: infrastructure development, political happenings and any other event that attracts public attention. Above all, helicopters have saved millions of lives across the world. I have worked shoulder to shoulder with people who have made this nation what it is today, especially in the underdeveloped frontiers along the Himalayas. I have spent nights in the exotic huts of tribals in Ladakh, Lahaul and Spiti, Arunachal Pradesh, Nagaland, Mizoram and Middle Andaman and Great Nicobar, among other places. They were truly priceless experiences.

When I started sharing some of my stories with my family and close friends, considerable disbelief was common. Friends who had rarely been out of metros, except for well-planned holidays abroad, could just not fathom the rich diversity their own country offered. Children loved my animal stories, and the aeroplanes and helicopters always excited them. Many young air warriors of my service are not aware of how life and work was managed far more frugally and fruitfully even without mobile phones or the internet!

My aim in penning down these stories is to bring out the diversity of India across its farthest corners, and also how life has changed over the decades in the air force in particular. While the 'lightness' and humour are intentional, in no way should it give the impression that a chopper pilot's job is less risky or less demanding. A 'good life' or a 'life well lived' may not have much to do with our bank balances or net worth, but it has everything to do with our diverse interactions in strange places with unfamiliar people. Those are the spices that make life's menu so tasty and nourishing.

## Dealing with Crazy A(H)erodynamics

Most people are confused as to how a bumblebee manages to fly, and that too quite well, against all odds. A helicopter is not too far down on the scale of people's consternation about oddities. It seems that such a seemingly unstable machine as a chopper is always about to crash—and it would too, if the pilot is not nimble enough. You can easily topple over if your wheel or skid lodges against something, and this can happen fast enough to surprise even a good pilot. This is called a dynamic rollover—how apt! There is an even more infamous and destructive phenomenon called ground resonance. This is akin to troops marching over a bridge in step, producing vibrations in sync with the natural frequency of the bridge. And voila, this resonance ultimately breaks the bridge. A chopper's oleo-pneumatic legs (landing gear) have a natural frequency, and a chopper is a huge vibrating object. You get the connect? This can cause complete destruction—and in just a few seconds!

A helicopter evolved from what was known as an autogyro, which had no tail rotor. It is the breakthrough of a tail rotor, which provides the counter torque to the main rotor, that has given a chopper its real capabilities. If not for this, a cockpit would rotate as fast as the main rotor in the opposite direction. But it brings with it a number of dangers and accidents waiting to happen. Many unsuspecting soldiers have walked into it in the heat of battle—and paid a heavy price with their limbs and lives. I was once captaining a sortie in Arunachal Pradesh, which involved 'hot' mission boarding of soldiers. While there are standard procedures and checks and balances, Murphy's Law ultimately prevails. My co-pilot was inside the cockpit, while I had jumped out to help the gunner ensure that no assault rifle was loaded live. And suddenly, out of the corner of my eye, I caught sight of a figure walking towards the tail rotor. I yelled amid the tremendous noise and din of the Mi-17, but before I knew it, he had walked right into the rotor, or rather, under it. I'm quite sure my crew and I missed a few heartbeats. This army captain happened to be the shortest officer I've ever met. He was a Gurkha and, thankfully, there are concessions on their minimum height during recruitment.

Of course, there was our 'Tail Rotor' Negi. He was an extremely accomplished and bold pilot with a great flying reputation who, later, narrowly escaped from the jaws of death. While doing a training sortie at night as a young pilot officer, he got off to do a crew change with the rotors running. He customarily started walking around the chopper and absent-mindedly went into the Chetak's tail rotor. Despite the shrieking noise of the fast-rotating rotor, he managed to do the unthinkable. He suffered some serious lacerations on his right arm, which put him down for about six months—but the name stuck.

A classic dynamic rollover leading to the complete wreck of a Mi-8 took place at a forward helipad in Sri Lanka. The Mi-8 was on the ground with rotors running and frenetic activity all around it. Suddenly, the captain heard a call from two light helicopters carrying the army's vice-chief, asking for some space. In a bid to oblige, and in the truest spirit of jointmanship, the Mi-8 captain hastened to shift to a corner of the large ground. Unfortunately, in doing so, while being too low, his main wheel struck a tree stump that was protruding but camouflaged naturally. And, before he realized it, the chopper tilted dangerously and crashed. The irony—the vice-chief did not manage to land!

We learnt about centre of gravity, or the C of G, in school long ago, with ample reiteration along the way. But the real lessons don't come home till you fly large aircraft or helicopters. At least the fixed-wing guys get trained people to load scientifically at most runways. Chopper guys do this at far-flung helipads with no weighing machines, and loaders with no education on the C of G or without a care in the world about its implications. It results in amusing and, sometimes, grave results. I was flying in Sri Lanka as part of the Indian Peace Keeping Force (IPKF) in a Mi-8. I was the captain while Kama was the co-pilot. We had landed in Talai Mannar, just off the beach, with the vast Indian Ocean in front, beckoning gently with its waves. In a hurry, and I suspect because of the wheeling and dealing of our flight gunner on ground (like changing currency!), who also doubles as load master, a quick offloading of supplies was done. Once the helicopter was offloaded, empty crates were to be put at the end of the cargo compartment first. But in the haste and the absence of the gunner in the compartment, all crates were piled up in the middle. Then in came the soldiers going back home. They got packed like sardines in the front half. The gunner came in last, not realizing what had happened. Quite evidently, the C of G was way forward and out of limits.

I got the go-ahead signal from my crew and picked up enough power to come to a hover. But 'she' suddenly pitched down and started taking off on her own. I had the stick fully back but to no avail. We barely skimmed the thankfully downward-sloping beach and reached the sea. Luckily, she had picked up enough speed to escape danger. A panicky five minutes of shifting crates and people followed, after which all was okay. But I never forgot the lessons of the C of G after that day. I hope my reference to an aircraft or helicopter in the feminine gender does not offend. It is an age-old pilot tradition. I am sure female pilots, who are equally capable, refer to their difficult-to-handle aircraft as a 'he'.

As if this is not enough of a headache, a chopper pilot (he or she) has to contend with the 3Ws—weight, weather and winds (not the more customary wine, women and song!). Each factor requires a separate book to cover all facets; however, the really dicey part is when any or all of them combine to present decision dilemmas to helicopter crews. A case in point is winds and their variability in strength and direction. Choppers are extremely sensitive to wind. Most performance graphs clearly highlight the beneficial effects of headwinds—you can actually carry far more with increasing headwinds. However, the downside of changing wind direction is normally ignored. The effects are exponentially worse since the tail rotor goes into a somewhat adverse performance regime. Tailwind is the worst in terms of its effects on load-lifting capacity and control in general. However, there are other directions, depending on the tail rotor's rotation and positioning, that can get you into a loss of tail rotor effectiveness. A number of helicopters have been lost due to inexplicable reasons (and conveniently attributed to human-error aircrew, or HE-A, while all the time it was loss of tail rotor effectiveness, or LTE. This has been well documented in the Russian handbook on aerodynamics for the Mi-25. In fact, there is no set template. Variances occur due to type, power requirements and the pilot's skills, among other reasons. Actually, in the Mi-25's case, any action by the pilot may aggravate the problem, so it's better to allow it to recover by itself!

The amount of weight you can carry depends on various factors, including winds, length of the helipad, slope for take-off or landing and the terrain in the approach funnel. It is easier to stick to the graphs or the unit standard operating procedures (SOPs), which give adequate safety margins. The problem starts when pilots (experienced ones too) put imaginary margins, or their own willpower, into the equation. A huge contributor to wrong practices in a helicopter landing at smaller helipads in the mountains is the skewed belief that a shallow approach is better when loaded up. Its origins can be traced back to the single-engine training at large helipads (up to 100 metres long), where a roller landing results from a shallow approach. This in turn is necessitated by low power margins. A corollary should be that shallow approaches should be done only when a roller landing is possible, meaning on larger helipads. However, the shallow approach is a no-go when there is turbulence, or wind shear, and when a roller-landing is not practical. There is an intricate balance of managing translational lift, collective (as a power tool and a decelerator) and inertia. If I've been able to confuse you, imagine what a chopper pilot has to deal with!

Weather, of course, is a problem with all pilots. But choppers have a context of inevitably flying closer to terrain, especially in the mountains and valleys. The urge to stay below clouds and manoeuvre is very strong, but so is the probability of controlled flight into terrain (CFIT)—as documented by hundreds of helicopter accidents. With newer and more capable machines and avionics, a sea change in approach is required. At the same time, operators should not bite off more than they can chew; it should be evolutionary and step-by-step. The first step would be for 'real' decision makers of macro policies to grasp the complexities and nuances of chopper operations.

We first came across the term 'dead man's curve' as rookie pilots. It was an area mapped on a height-versus-speed graph that did not allow safe recovery from an engine failure. It scared the wits out of us initially. As the years passed, and hours under the belt increased, fear and respect were replaced by a fatalistic 'it can't happen to me'. No wonder this term has now been replaced the world over by 'avoid area'. Most chopper pilots are always on the edge, waiting for the worst to happen. There have been innumerable bar discussions on whether this ultimately reflects on our life philosophy! I once heard an old retired chopper pilot, who never rose beyond the rank of a wing commander (equal to a lieutenant colonel), say that rising in his career was not half as relevant as making it out alive at the end of it. It is true—the fatality rates of helicopter pilots in action are the highest among all in non-war conditions. No wonder they have the highest number of gallantry awards to their credit.

The IAF's helicopter fleet history has been captured as a snapshot at the end of this book as an epilogue. I have deliberately done that because it is a legacy that is to be appreciated. Since this book is about humorously told stories that happen to most chopper pilots, I did not want to mix anything into this flavour. The full history of the IAF's helicopter fleet is documented in my book *The Purple Legacy*.

The first helicopter in the world was the VS-300. Igor Sikorsky, who developed it, famously said, 'It would be safe to say that the helicopter's role in saving lives represents one of the most glorious pages in the history of human flight. If a man is in need of rescue, an airplane can come in and throw flowers on him, and that's just about all. But a direct lift aircraft could come in and save his life.'

# STRANGER THAN FICTION

# STRANGE ENCOUNTERS

ALL THE STORIES in this section are about animals and the hilarious outcomes of their meetings with humans in general, and pilots in particular. Watching nature in full bloom makes you wonder why most humans are so hesitant to embrace diversity. It can bring so much colour, creativity and joy to life. These tales are about real encounters with snakes, dogs, man-eaters, mithuns (a cross between wild gaurs and domestic cattle) and many others across the country. They also try to bring out the richness of life in military cantonments.

This section is a vast canvas covering the icy heights of Ladakh and moving to the lush and thick jungles of Arunachal Pradesh. From pets to savage wild animals, chopper pilots encounter all during their duty. Some stories also paint our sometimes-inept handling of them, which result in unintended and humorous episodes. Truly, life is stranger than fiction—and we should thank our stars for that!

## An Early Start

### East Pakistan Trauma

My association with the IAF started way back in 1972. My dad was in the Indian Foreign Service. We had come back to India in October 1971, just before the Indo-Pak War. Our otherwise blissful time of three years in Dacca (now Dhaka) included the almost eight months we spent under house arrest by the Pakistani army. This included the full high commission with families. All of us were confined to a multistorey complex in Kakrail, with only one officer allowed to go with a coolie to Shanti Bazaar, once a week, to shop for the whole community. No school, no outings, and yet we kids made the most of it. All of us were evacuated by two planes of Swissair and Aeroflot one fine day, sans any luggage. Everyone lost everything. We saw it all from our windows and roofs of the six-storey building.

Our kids' gang had adopted a puppy that was half-dead when we picked it up from a field. We named it—no surprise here—Tommy. Fed by almost every household in the building, it grew up fast and strong. He was a terror for all outsiders but a darling to all occupants. I can never forget that night when we were being whisked away to the airport, with Tommy chasing our vans for many miles and all of us weeping away. My mom told us that he came up to the airport! For many years, I wondered what became of Tommy. Finally, we got the answer after decades, from an officer who went back after the 1971 war. Tommy found his way back to the building. Our landlord's kids looked after him, even though he didn't eat for many days after we left.

I witnessed the genocide first-hand as a child, along with others in the building complex: the horror of killings at point-blank range, the screaming of women being gang-raped, naked men being paraded and forced to crawl on the hot asphalt roads, all done in public view to intimidate and instil fear. The worst was the massacre at Shanti Bazaar. One fine Sunday, there was a big commotion in the building and everyone went up to the roof. One could see the huge marketplace in the distance, which used to be packed on Sundays. A few fire engines had gathered along with armed forces in huge numbers, with vehicles mounted with machine guns. In an orchestrated move, all exits of Shanti Bazaar were blocked just when it was most crowded. And then the ring of shops that surrounded it were set on fire and people running away were fired at. The fire engines stopped the fire from expanding to unintended places. Later in life, during history lessons at school, I would compare it with the massacre at Jallianwala Bagh.

The only thing that we were allowed to carry back to India was my little sister's (three years then) doll, which was taller than her. On landing at Palam airport in Delhi, at a ground reception, my sister and her doll became the star attraction of news reporters—she was there on all front covers the next day along with the horror stories that families related. Many years later, my parents told us that it was a touch-and-go situation with each day full of uncertainty about whether we would survive or not.

## 'Centralian' Canopy

Now, back to the subject of the beginnings of my long association with the IAF. Air Force Central School, or AFCS in New Delhi's Subroto Park, subsequently renamed The Air Force School (TAFS), was the starting point. My dad had to put me in the hostel since he was leaving for Belgium in fifteen days. So there I was, in July 1972, in an IAF school from a completely non-military background—nobody in my extended family had ever thought about the military except for the 'Jai Jawan Jai Kisan' sloganeering. Actually, AFCS had no visible mark of being a 'military' school. It was a proper public school with the majority of students coming from a civilian background. Under a legendary principal, Hari Dang, the school was rated as one of the best. Mr Dang worked tirelessly to give his students a holistic education, including sports, co-curricular activities, wildlife excursions and everything else. We were major participants in the Duke of Edinburgh's Award scheme, which was later renamed the President's Award Programme.

I remember August 1972, when the school received a war trophy—a Pakistani tank from the Battle of Longewala. The whole day was spent watching this mammoth being mounted on a hump. I also remember the many years we spent fighting mock battles, and some other pleasant memories with girlfriends, around this tank! The school had a house system with five inspiring names—Jagriti, Shakti, Jyoti, Kirti and Shanti. Aravalli Lodge, the hostel for over 200 students, was a hotbed of inter-house rivalry from the sports fields to Holi or Diwali fights. The serene house names had no bearing on this 'healthy' rivalry. But like most school hostels, it imbibed confidence, self-belief and fiery competitiveness in most.

But there were exceptions. Shahid Ali , the grandson of famous ornithologist Dr Salim Ali, was two batches my senior. He was soft-spoken, reticent and a decent boy—a slight misfit in the rough crowd. But he had a special talent for which he was well respected, and also given the farthest and corner-most room to himself. I forget the number of snakes and reptiles he kept in it! He even had a python at the Delhi Zoo. He got it for display on one Founder's Day at school. In the interim, he kept it in the principal's bathroom, from where it slithered off into the adjoining staffroom. There was pandemonium and public displays of emotion that amply demonstrated which of our teachers had guts.

Our school campus was infested with snakes—mostly kraits, vipers and cobras. It was not unusual for hostelers to kill one when they discovered one in the buildings. It was also quite normal to see Shahid dashing—rare as it was—to save the snake. He was an absolute expert at catching and handling them gently.

Our annual sojourns to Corbett National Park during the Dussehra holidays were a high point for me. The enjoyable bus rides spent singing songs at our loudest, our stories of animal encounters, and campfires deep inside Corbett are all beautiful memories of our annual tryst with nature. Our usual mentor for these was A.K. Singh, our PT teacher. A short and well-muscled man, he was actually a wrestler of repute. All the boys used to hole up in one room and the girls in another. AK and his family used to stay in a small cottage some fifty metres away. One dark night, we had just gone into our sleeping bags when the conversation turned to AK. There were loud guffaws and everyone came up with 'AK' jokes, some definitely below the belt. Suddenly, one of us identified a bear-like silhouette on the fly-proof door and yelled, 'Oh god, a bhalu [bear] is outside!' Pat came the reply, 'It's me, you ***. Go to sleep or I'll eat you all up.' There wasn't a peep from any of us after that.

## Snakes in the Cockpit

### Hakimpet Horror

This story is from Hakimpet, near Hyderabad, where fledgling helicopter pilots take their first baby steps. One afternoon an odd emergency cropped up. A Chetak helicopter had just taken off, but had abruptly landed in front of the air traffic control on the taxi-track. The call by the pilots was panicky and garbled; however, the word 'cobra' was clearly heard.

A cobra that had somehow found its way into the passenger cabin and was sleeping peacefully was induced to slide forward, since a chopper takes off with an excessive nose-down attitude. It went unnoticed till it raised its hood in response to the instructor's foot movement. Hakimpet witnessed the fastest landing, switch-off and pilot exit ever at that time! A similar incident happened to me in 1984 while flying in the Northeast.

## Mizoram Menace

I was doing a detachment with a Chetak helicopter in Aizawl, Mizoram, in 1985. The army had constructed a small hangar next to Zemabawk helipad, with two rooms to serve as workstations for the air and ground crews. Those were the days of heightened insurgency across the states of Tripura, Mizoram, Nagaland and Assam, and we had to fly all across with multiple agencies involved in counter-insurgency and supporting governance. Life was frugal and full of hardships in every sense; albeit with a high sense of accomplishment.

Air navigation was rudimentary, with voluminous 'quarter-inch' maps that detailed contours, and was completely reliant on a pilot's skills to read them. A 'moving-thumbs' display was the surest navigation aid, where a pilot's fingers or thumb tracked the helicopter movement on the map by the minute. It meant carrying huge bundles or folds of maps that were neatly covered with plastic sheets. These were put under the passenger seats for use during the flight.

One fine morning, we took off early for Agartala in Tripura. The schedule was to pick up the director general (DG) of the Border Security Force (BSF) and three other senior officers who were to arrive from Delhi, give them an aerial survey of two hours over some areas mapped out and land at a base called Bogafa for the DG's detailed briefing and lunch. Post-lunch, after dropping the team back at Agartala, we were to head back to Aizawl.

The sortie (mission) went as planned till Bogafa. After landing, we closed all the doors so that nobody would tamper with the control systems out of curiosity. We were to wait in the officer's mess for the DG and his team for the elaborate lunch. But only half an hour later, a constable came running to us—we were required at the helipad urgently. Now, Bogafa helipad was a small football ground with not a blade of grass on the hard-baked mud surface. On reaching there, we discovered quite a commotion around our helicopter, with at least a dozen BSF soldiers on alert with lathis. A captain-equivalent BSF officer explained that a green snake was inside the chopper. We briefed the soldiers on what not to do and opened the cargo doors. Within no time they had killed the snake, which turned out to be a green pit viper of the poisonous variety.

We soundly rebuked all and sundry present, but secretly wondered how the slippery passenger had managed to get inside a locked chopper after traversing a large baked-clay football field. The mystery was solved in Aizawl. Our ground crew, on hearing of a snake in the helicopter, inquired whether it was green in colour. It emerged that a day ago, they had spotted it in the pilot's room and, despite their best efforts, they could not track it, assuming in the end that it had escaped. Quite obviously, it had hidden in the maps and was comfortable till the helicopter heated up at Bogafa!

## Homely Herpetons

A helicopter pilot of the IAF gets posted to some of the most cut-off, quaint and least developed regions of the country. The good part is that though the families rough it out, they get a chance to be together even in hard field areas—albeit on the quiet in non-family stations. In 1988, I was posted from Jaisalmer in Rajasthan to Car Nicobar in the Andamans. My wife, Sheel, joined me with our two children after six months. My daughter was two years old then and my son just six months old. Our house was a temporary one-room outfit with a veranda covered with tin sheets, which served as a kitchen. The sea was just twenty metres away and the atmosphere was out of this world. Life was good with uniquely challenging operations at sea in Russian Mi-8 helicopters—an ample variety ranging from anti-piracy, civilian inter-island support, joint operations with the navy, to name just a few.

As a young flight lieutenant, I was told to look after the officer's mess, which was about 2 km from home. An official reception for a visiting air marshal was scheduled for one night and I was immersed in protocol and other arrangements. There was only one landline phone in our domestic cluster. The mess incharge came up to me and told me that a snake had been discovered in my house. I immediately took permission and ran the 2 km, picking up an IAF policeman from the guardroom on the way. It turned out that Sheel had gone to the makeshift kitchen and found a 'long' piece of cloth hanging from the top at one corner. Closer scrutiny showed that it was a reticulated python (15 feet, as measured later) whose both ends were still not visible. The tail was outside while the head was behind the cooking range and fridge. She had bolted the door to our room and requested a neighbour who was at home to help. Not knowing what to do, he had decided to get the master of the house quickly on the scene!

The kitchen had space for just one person to enter, and I had hoped the police corporal would know what to do. He declined but held up a thick stick to help out. I had to go in. The snake was nowhere in sight, so I got on my knees with a torch while the corporal watched from the doorway. Suddenly, the python's head appeared behind me, from under the cooking range, of which I was blissfully unaware. The supercharged corporal let out a war cry and some expletives in Malayalam and struck at least ten blows to the python's head. The snake died there and then, without a chance for us to shoo it out somehow, which I had hoped to do. While measuring it, we ran out of length on the tailoring tape and had to use a foot ruler.

## More at Home

Zora, our white boxer, was a very demanding member of the family. She was hyper, did not listen to any instructions that did not promise food in the end and was the darling of the kids. But during our posting at Hindon airbase, she proved her worth—in a way that the family still remembers fifteen years after her death.

We had a ground floor house with an attached room that housed the electrical junction box. Full of the usual administration junk, it was basically no one's baby; it just served as a rat colony. I was an air force examiner and was in office debriefing my boss, the commanding officer (CO), on my last inspection. The children were at school. The CO's phone rang; he listened intently and then asked me to hurry with my report. I did so in the next ten minutes, after which he ordered me to rush home since a cobra had been spotted there. I zipped back as fast as possible along with my colleague and fellow examiner, Pannu.

The story was that Sheel had gone out for a ladies' club meeting, locking Zora inside the house. When she returned, she could hear Zora barking away even before she had entered the driveway. On opening the main door, she found Zora all over the sofa in front of the door to the electrical room. She was furiously sniffing, barking incessantly and leaping up and down from the sofa—all at the same time. My wife did not see anything, so she tied Zora to the handle of the main door. Zora continued barking even after my wife changed and came back out. That's when she noticed a thick black snake slithering out from under the sofa towards the bedroom. Each time it came out, Zora would bark and charge towards it, restrained by the long leash. This would send it back. Sheel picked up a stick and kept banging it on the floor to ensure that the snake did not slither out. At the same time, she phoned my office.

Pannu and I finally killed the poor snake, not knowing what else to do in that moment. It was a six-foot-long, fully grown cobra, known for its deadly venom. After that, we never criticized our loveable but hyper dog, knowing that she had saved us from what could have been a dangerous situation.

## Even More!

I once watched a BBC documentary that debated the chances of getting a snakebite inside of a WC pot (toilet). I think it was one in a few million. But I almost defied this statistic on two occasions. The first was during a family holiday from the airbase at Mohanbari to Along in the mountains of Arunachal Pradesh. Traversing the mighty Brahmaputra on a ferry, across its multiple channels, took a full day, so we spent the night at the army camp at Likabali. Single-line barracks had been converted into a guest accommodation with two rooms and an attached bathroom at the end. We tucked in early since the next day's drive was a long one, through a thousand mountain curves.

I woke up at 5 a.m. to finish my ablutions before waking up the family. There was no electricity since the generators would come on only at 6 a.m. With a torch I found my way to the toilet, flashed it around for safety and almost sat on the WC. But something caught my eye even in the dim light. I pointed the torch into the WC, and lo and behold, a krait, an extremely venomous variety, was squirming around before it disappeared into the sewer pipe. Despite frantic efforts by the army jawans to locate it, it could not be found. Finally, some kerosene was flushed down to ensure the WC was safe to use. I kept quiet about it since there was no other toilet around except for the common one in the soldiers' barracks some distance away. My family heard about this only when we were halfway to Along—anyway, they did not believe me!

A decade later, I was commanding the Helicopter Training School at Hyderabad. While a completely new block had come up for training and administration; for the sake of tradition and legacy, the CO's office was still in an older block adjoining the hangar that housed all the helicopters. My routine included an early-morning check on maintenance activities around sunrise, going back home (some 8 km away) and then getting back to office around 8.30 a.m. when flying was on in full swing.

One day, I found some commotion outside my office. The janitor told me that a small snake had been found on the WC. The whole bathroom and my office were given a thorough shake-up before normal work resumed. The snake was sent for identification. The next day, it was the same routine, including the commotion outside my office. Another snake had been found at almost the same spot, now identified as a 'sapola' or a fledgling cobra. A fire tender was called in to flush out the entire sewage pipe system that was underground. The people on duty at the exit point counted twenty-seven sapolas that were flushed out. Thus the theory that someone was conspiring against the CO (me) was negated and the blame was put squarely on the 'nagin' that had left her clutch of eggs in an inconvenient place!

### Tambaram Twister

The strangest thing happened in Tambaram, Madras (now Chennai), where I had gone to train as an instructor at the Flying Instructors School (FIS). The schedule was heavy for all five months, with the only saving grace being that families were allowed to rough it out together in a one-room accommodation. Flying was in two shifts, forenoon and later, with two squadrons alternating weekly. To and fro travel was done on our motorcycles since it allowed some flexibility at pack-up, which, depending on your FIS instructor, varied from early evening to late night. Helmets were compulsory while riding and were generally left on the motorcycles. Chennai is part of Romulus Whitaker's (a famous herpetologist) forest range of the most prolific venomous snakes. In fact, Chennai houses a famous snake park set up by the equally famous naturalist.

One day, just before noon, my co-pupil Vashist and I picked up our bikes and set off to FIS with me trailing behind him. At the midpoint (a guardroom), a police sergeant initially gave us the signal to pass but on coming closer, he gesticulated wildly for us to stop. Vashist found the sergeant keeping his distance but repeatedly pointing at his helmet. Vashist took it off and almost immediately threw it away on discovering a snake in it. Imagine the sergeant's surprise when he saw an officer riding by with a snake's head protruding from his helmet. This is exactly how Lord Shiva is depicted! After that, all trainee officers not only checked their bikes and helmets, but in general kept a good look-out at home for these critters as well.

## Save the Snake!

Among all these hair-raising near-misses, there were many cases of fatal snakebites too, especially at night. A colleague lost his wife to a cobra bite. The diagnosis took time since only one pin-prick was seen on the big toe. Unfortunately, her condition deteriorated rapidly until it was too late. Incidentally, the other fang of the cobra was discovered embedded in her bathroom slippers later. Mare, my flight commander in the Congo peacekeeping mission, just about survived a lethal cobra bite at Jammu. All this brings me to one common observation, which is not actually a real Eureka moment. Snakes come where rats and frogs thrive; cleaning up your house and surroundings may solve half the problem. Now I get it—the logic of pre-Diwali cleaning and even Swachh Bharat!

## Save the Bitten!

A particularly memorable snakebite evacuation that I did in Aizawl, Mizoram, comes to mind. I had just landed at the mandatory last landing at sunset with the top General on board when his Colonel, looking after operations, approached the helicopter whose rotors were still running. He came up to me and pointed towards a mountain across the river (Dhaleshwari), to an army post called Riek. A Gurkha jawan had been bitten on the head by a viper. The only possible evacuation on foot would take at least thirty-six hours, and the doctors did not think he would survive for more than a few hours. Air evacuation was the only way out. However, since it was past last landing, I went through a five-minute decision dilemma. There was only a landline to the chief of operations (COO) at the faraway base of Kumbhirgram near Silchar, and it would take at least thirty minutes to get through to him. Night flying was prohibited since these were times when one had not even heard of night-vision devices.

I took the call as only a young flying officer would, with little knowledge and even lesser fear of ramifications. Disembarking the General, I flew to Riek with instructions to light up the helipad with everything possible. One look at the soldier being brought on a stretcher convinced me of having done the right thing. His head was swollen and grotesque—like an alien from another planet. After landing in Aizawl, I got through to the COO at Kumbhirgram base. The next fifteen minutes were spent in listening to the choicest expletives and details of my extremely objectionable professional conduct and poor pedigree. He could not ground me since there was no other captain to fly the next day. The soldier did survive, which was very gratifying; however, the written warning a few days later was not. But that's aviation for you—hot and cold, and unpredictable.

## Animals Versus Pilots!

### Hashi Hathis

My first operational posting as a pilot officer was to Hashimara in West Bengal, along its border with Assam. Except for the runway, the entire base was covered in dense forest that stood out like a sore thumb among the acres of cultivated land for miles around. Jaldapara Sanctuary was about 50 km away, and this stretch must have been part of the ancient trail of elephant herds that once roamed freely. As a result, a regular feature was the appearance of elephants during seasons coinciding with certain harvests.

If you were to ask any old-timer at Hashimara, he would swear by the fact that these massive but gentle giants stuck to the forests and had never damaged any worthwhile air force assets. However, in 1983, it was ordained differently. I remember the excitement of the just-formed 'Thunderbolts' aerobatic team and their daily practice over the base. The base commander, a veteran fighter pilot of the 1971 war fame, and his advisers decided that something had to be done about this pachyderm problem. While sightings were reported from the forests, one incident involved a uniformed guard who had fired a shot in the air to frighten a herd, which he could just about discern in the forests. An enraged matriarch had pulled down his makeshift chowkidar machan. He had, of course, run away as the herd approached.

A count revealed seventeen elephants in the herd, including some young ones. The advice of old-timers was to let it go, but to no avail. The herd was tracked and disturbed to shoo them away, but the forests were too thick and it remained cohesive. A war room was activated and minds got together to 'solve' the problem. It was finally decided that a helicopter would be used to shoo them away. So, on the third day after the first sighting, my flight commander took me along for some fun flying. We located the herd in the middle of the thick forest. Every trick in the book, including low passes, mock dives and even direct hovering over them, was tried. I wasn't even aware that a helicopter could be so manoeuvrable! At the end of an hour, the herd had dispersed and disappeared. Mighty satisfied, we returned as saviours. But the halo was short-lived.

While earlier the herd was always sighted together, now reports came in of multiple small herds and solitary elephants from virtually all over the station. Desperate to find each other, they went on a rampage wherever challenged. Everything came to a stop for the next few days, including the Thunderbolts. Finally, the forest department at Jaldapara was consulted. Following their advice, the herd was not disturbed any further, some damage was tolerated and the herd was allowed to gather and leave after a few days. The pachyderms had done more damage in a few days than what they had managed to do in the last two decades. Incidentally, the elephants returned over the next two years that I was there. But now the commanders of Hashimara were wiser!

## Tootsie

My first dog after joining the IAF, Tootsie, was a golden Lhasa apso from the King of Bhutan's royal kennel. I was privileged to fly the king's sisters and others over a few days. The king was not allowed in a single-engine helicopter. When His Highness asked if he could do anything for me, I requested for a pup. Like every mountain dog, Tootsie was extremely temperamental and forever in a fight with me as to who was the boss. I was a Dustin Hoffman fan, and therefore the name; as also the fact that you could never make out which side was the head and which the tail!

It was a mistake to own a pet as a bachelor. With so many moves and detachments at faraway places like Guwahati and Aizawl, it was impossible to take Tootsie along in a service helicopter. However, in the winter of 1984, I was asked to move to Aizawl the next day. No one agreed to care for a loveable but temperamental pet. There was just no way I could find anyone to look after Tootsie. I did the unthinkable—packed him in a carton with holes and took him along in the chopper. At the intermediate halt for refuelling at Shillong, I managed to pull off a hoodwinking act with those present and took him out to do his job. Finally, we were at Aizawl with all its freedom. Our *sahayak,* or helper, became very fond of Tootsie, and he became the darling of all the army soldiers and officers who were with us.

Tootsie also used to accompany us to the helipad, where he was free to roam around under watchful eyes. I did notice a lot of locals (Mizos) who would turn up to admire him, and the crowd kept getting bigger as the days passed. It was only after a few days that a local friend of mine, Zoramthanga, warned me about taking care of my pet. Perplexed, I asked him what was wrong. He in turn queried, 'Have you seen any dog for miles around?' I realized that this observation was true—there were no dogs around. Why? Because among some tribes, dog meat is a favourite! On the very next helicopter going back, I took Tootsie to the safety of Hashimara. The only dogs around in the hundreds of helipads in Mizoram and Nagaland were those kept as sentry dogs by the army and Border Security Force. They gave early warning of arriving locals or insurgents.

### Thoise Troubles

My entire family adores dogs and swears by the loyalty of man's best friend. However, I will relate two incidents that happened in Ladakh, which taught me to be slightly circumspect. As a young flight lieutenant, I used to be deployed for detachments at Thoise in the Nubra Valley, beyond the famed Khardung La Pass. Winters there were truly harsh with temperatures plummeting to as low as -25 degrees Celsius, and even lower when the wind-chill factor was considered. We used to stay in temporary sheds-cum-mud constructions. In fact, prefabricated huts with insulation had just arrived on the scene—the initial ones were reserved for senior functionaries. Like all such forward bases, the place had a large strength of local dogs (mastiffs and hybrids) that usually waited for scraps and slept in the sun by day. Our days used to end early. Dinner was finished one hour after sunset, with heavy drinkers taking a little more time. Do remember that one had to get up early to prepare the helicopters in sub-zero temperatures. First take-offs were at sunrise, with the sun still hidden in the mountains for another hour. Life was tough but very satisfying while actively supporting the battle for the Siachen Glacier. In the old days, there were quite a few heavy drinkers, but then we were blissfully ignorant; unlike today, where medical science and our doctors have more than caught up with the latest on alcohol-related issues.

One morning in the winter of 1990, some airmen going towards the helicopters in the dark discovered a half-eaten body of a junior warrant officer. He had alcohol dependence syndrome (ADS) and had probably had one too many that night. While walking back alone, he saw a pack of about twenty dogs that magically congregated when humans went to sleep. In his stupor, he threw a stone at the pack, which was not really interested in him. We got to know this later from one of his friends who recounted that he had thrown stones at them earlier as well, going by his boasts at the bar. But that night, the pack attacked him and due to scarcity of food, ate half of his body. As far as I remember, it never happened again for decades.

After almost twenty years, I was back at Leh airbase as the commander. Seeing a large number of stray dogs at the station, my lessons from the yesteryears served to motivate me to address the situation. I needed help from the adjoining engineer force (GREF), so I met the commanding officer. He consulted his camp and politely declined, saying that they had coexisted for years without any problem. Anyway, I did my bit to ensure aircraft operations in Leh were not compromised.

The IAF's IL-76, a large-bodied aeroplane, is colloquially called 'IL-Baba' in winters since it is the lifeline of Ladakh when all roads and passes close. We used to start a small vegetable shop on a no-profit-no-loss basis for the villagers around. The menu that night, or the next day, depended on whether IL-Baba came in or not. Villagers would make a beeline for the shop. One day, a GREF labourer's family sent their thirteen-year-old daughter to stand in the line for some vegetables. Her house was barely 100 metres away but through a narrow 'gali' or lane. By the time she started back, darkness had fallen; there was snow all around and it was cold. No one heard any commotion in their homes because of noisy bukharis, charcoal or fuel-based heating devices, running at their full capacity. And anyway, dogs would fight among themselves every night.

When the girl did not return till 9 p.m., a search was launched for her. At the air force gate, which closed much earlier, the crowd was told that no civilian was inside. After some searching, they discovered a pack of dogs that was still eating her. These were the same strays that infested the entire area every day. The next day, a sad commanding officer of the GREF came to me to apologize. In the next few days, they exterminated almost twenty dogs, not realizing that as long as food refuse or waste was available, they would thrive and multiply. One had to be careful at night in the harsh winters of Leh.

## Bachiya and a Man-Eating Tiger

I love the mountains and none compare to our own majestic Himalayas. There is an entire range of wooded hills beneath the highest mountains in the world—full of flora and fauna of great diversity. While at school in TAFS, I always volunteered for the autumn excursions to Corbett National Park or the Kumaon hills. This love remains till date. I have read everything ever written by Jim Corbett and consider him an icon of courage and compassion with regard to wild animals. Man-eating fears are quite natural for people just initiated into jungles. It takes awareness and knowledge to realize how rare man-eaters are and why some big cats turn into them.

In 1986, I had gone on a long rafting camp on the Ganges while training for an expedition on River Zanskar. The camp was opposite Shivpuri village in Uttarakhand, through which the highway passed. On reaching Shivpuri, we used to ferry across by rafts to the campsite. Tigers and leopards were regular sightings from this side, especially if one had patience. It was heaven—hard work in the early mornings, rafting and practice up to Rishikesh till noon and then idyllic relaxation till sunset with a campfire before turning in early for the night.

One day, we had a visitor from Delhi—a Mr Menon working in the defence ministry, quite obviously on a leisure trip. He came across in the early evening but seemed to be crest-fallen and quite ashen-faced. While waiting for the raft at Shivpuri, he claimed to have clearly heard the villagers say that a tiger had lifted a bachcha, or child, the previous night. He had inquired again and the villagers had repeated, '*Bagh bachcha utha le gaya.*' He had actually decided to go back, but no vehicle was available. We had no way to confirm this, and suddenly the thought of tiger sightings became a threat. That night, the campfire would not end since no one wanted to leave the group for the tents, which were a little further away. A luxury tent had been erected for Menon, but he insisted on sleeping in my tent. You can imagine the sleepless night; loud coughs and torch flashes ensued all through.

The next morning, a headcount showed all in, including Menon. There was a big hurry to get across and speak to the people of the village. The mystery got resolved in a jiffy. A tiger had lifted a calf, or *bachra* (in local dialect '*bachiya*'). The 'ch' in bachcha and bachiya are distinctive to Hindi-speaking people. But Menon, who was from south India, picked up on what he feared most in his heart and heard 'bachcha'. The result was a sleepless night for all of us, but the great relief afterwards more than made up for it. However, Menon left the same day.

## Mohanbari Musings

The helicopter base at Dibrugarh, Upper Assam, is known to the IAF as Mohanbari, named after a small village adjoining the base. With its mighty Mi-17 helicopters, this base has been a pillar of support in war and peace in the Northeast, particularly in Assam and Arunachal Pradesh. The logo of the base is a snarling leopard amid forests and tea gardens. In 1942, huge forests were cleared to construct the base. It was initially called Lahoal Air Force Base. As with many airfields in the India's Northeast, World War II operations saw the airfield very busy with cargo-carrying trips over the hump to Burma and China. After Independence, Mohanbari was instrumental in creating an air bridge to the most forward areas of the Northeast. Leopards still did the rounds and it was not unusual in the 1980s–90s to come across them. There is a popular belief that leopards love dog meat. There is an even more popular story of an officer named Gill, whose pet (Rani) was once chased by a leopard in the evening on a road between the officers' houses.

The only thing that saved the dog was Gill chasing right behind, yelling at the top of his voice! Old friends who were there at that time swear by this story. Till date, that road is known as Leopard Lane.

When I was a CO there in early 2000, I used to go for my weekend runs along the 'kutcha' perimeter road. On at least eight occasions, I spotted pug marks and twice, a leopard. One evening, the station commander came around collecting all the children playing in the park for a free leopard sighting tour. A call had come in from a sentry regarding this. From a distance of about 150 metres, this noisy bunch watched two leopards (a mother and an almost fully grown cub) playing near the perimeter wall. The mother was sitting on the wall while the youngster was frolicking in the grass, oblivious to all the commotion. Suddenly, the commander grabbed the sentry's rifle and fired an aimed shot. Thankfully, it hit the wall between the two animals. In a flash, they disappeared into the adjoining tea gardens. It was only later that realization dawned that had he hit either of them, he would have committed a crime. His excuse till date is that he aimed between them!

## Majestic Mithuns

Mithuns, which are a cross between wild gaur and domestic cattle, are revered all over India's Northeast. Among the many tribes of Arunachal Pradesh, such as the Mishmis and Apatanis, they are a symbol of wealth and well-being and a must as dowry to the bride's side. They are actually semi-wild, as I found out to my dismay.

I was on a squadron trek from Hayuliang on River Lohit to Chakla Gaon towards the Chinese border. It was an arduous six-day trek along a narrow track through steep mountains that were heavily forested. Only one person could be on this track with vertical downward slopes on one side and thickly vegetated upward slopes on the other. We had started as a six-member team, but by the fourth day, only two of us were left since the others had fallen sick and were left behind at Border Road Organization set-ups. The purpose of the trek was to identify potential areas to be cleared for helipads to support road-building efforts by air.

The going was tough and we were looking forward to reaching our destination, which was another camp just one day away from Chakla Gaon. We had been warned of the presence of leeches, especially the havildar leech that was famous among army soldiers. They were so named because of the three sergeant-like yellow stripes that ran along their bodies when they were full of blood. As we turned a bend, I stopped abruptly as, right in front of me, about 15 feet away, was a mithun occupying the entire space. Panic subsided when we realized that the animal was absolutely 'chilled out', with no movement except for an occasional swish of the tail. It gave an aura of calmness, infinite patience and, of course, a sturdy resolve to have his way. After about ten minutes, we realized that the only ones that needed to give way was us. The slope towards the valley was too steep and dangerous, while the upwards slope was slippery with no solid branches to hold on to. Anyway, after some effort, we managed to crawl up on all fours and hang on to whatever vegetation we could. But the giant would not move. After an interminable half an hour, the beast finally moved. It ambled below us in slow motion, as if to rub in the insult even more. We got down after it passed. It was massive and may have weighed more than a tonne.

On reaching our destination, the first cup of tea was heavenly, until something dropped out of my windcheater sleeve. It was a fully bloated havildar leech. On further examination, and a lot of salt and cigarette treatment later, we counted about twenty of them between the two of us. All of them had crawled in when we were clutching at the leaves on the upslope. Quite obviously, our mithun had the proverbial last laugh.

## Something Fishy

In Latin, India means the country of the River Indus. The mighty Indus flows majestically through a wide valley where Leh is nestled. As a helicopter pilot, I had been associated with the river since 1987, when a rafting camp was held here. I had come from Jaisalmer in Rajasthan to a new kind of desert. Since then, I have flown various helicopters in Ladakh, but the beauty of the Indus remained unsurpassable. Swimming in the cold waters seems to truly cleanse one of all mental stress, if not 'paap'.

There is abundant fish in the river, especially mountain trout. However, the rainbow trout, a delicacy served in Leh restaurants, is not from the local river but from Manali in Himachal Pradesh. I got to know the reason a few decades later, when I commanded the airbase at Leh. No one fishes in the stretch of the Indus that flows through Leh valley. Not only is it a national park (Hemis), but the fish are also considered sacred by certain Buddhist sects. According to some locals, as part of religious rites, when a person from one of these sects dies, the body is cut up into many parts, prayed to and then offered to the river and its fishes. That is why no one eats these fishes. However, way downstream, around Kargil, there is considerable fishing of mountain trout.

During the same rafting camp in 1987, we used to start driving east to Hemis before sunrise, raft down crossing abeam Leh, and finally stop at Nimu where the Indus and Zanskar meet. While driving back from Nimu to Leh, we invariably stopped at the famous Sikh shrine of Pathar Sahib for langar. Guru Nanak Dev, the founder of the Sikh religion, is said to have visited this spot. While meditating below a hill, a demon had tried to kill him by nudging a large boulder downhill. The stone, however, had stopped just short of Guru Nanak Dev. 'Pathar' means stone in Hindi, which is why the shrine is called Pathar Sahib. Through the decades, every soldier and regiment deployed in these areas pays obeisance here and offers seva.

## Deity Name Change

Much later, when I was air officer commanding (AOC) in Leh, some locals gave me an alternative version of the story. It turns out that until India's independence, this story was attributed to a Buddhist monk and spiritual leader. However, after Leh was saved by the Indian Army in 1947, flying in Dakotas piloted by the courageous gang led by IAF's Baba Mehar Singh—a Sikh himself—the population increased manifold mainly due to the arrival of the armed forces' units. And the myths and beliefs also grew.

According to an article in the *Indian Express*[*] in 2020, there is an explanation for the gurdwara there. During the construction of the Leh–Nimu road in the late 1970s, a large boulder with Buddhist prayer flags tied to it was found in the middle of the road. A lot of attempts were made to move the boulder from there, but everything failed, including bulldozers that were brought in. Many say that that night, some locals dreamt that a higher force was telling them not to move the boulder—and so it stayed. The Sikh regiment of the Indian Army, with the help of the locals, built the gurdwara at that very spot, with the boulder incorporated within its premises. Whatever be the truth, it is a much-cherished destination for all tourists visiting Leh.

A similar story seems to have evolved in the Spituk Monastery, next to the airbase at Leh. From there you can watch airplanes land. Within this complex is a Kali Mandir that has mainly Buddhist paintings and murals all around it. Even the idols are distinctly of Buddhist or Tibetan origin.

---

* Divya A., 'Why Guru Nanak Stayed in Leh', *The Indian Express*, 2 February 2020, https://indianexpress.com/article/express-sunday-eye/why-guru-nanak-stayed-in-leh-6242839/lite/

There is also a small Shiva Mandir on the Indus, close to Spituk, that gets submerged whenever the river overflows. It is a great picnic spot with the most breathtaking views. If you spend the day there, you will notice the mountains, sky, river and everything else change colours and hues all the time. It is truly mesmerizing. An island across has a forest full of stunted trees, as if somebody had attempted bonsai. Ladakhi ponies, which are semi-wild, rule the island and even charged at me when I attempted to explore it once.

## Jai Bajrangi

Hanuman, India's favourite god, is worshipped with fervour all over. He stands for devotion, integrity, commitment and strength—all desirable qualities in combatants—which explains his presence at every temple in our bases. A spin-off is the respect accorded to monkeys (his Vanar Sena or monkey army) everywhere. It also translates into a great menace because of the destruction caused by them—and killing them is considered a sin. The chief culprit is the common rhesus monkey. Airbases have almost become helpless, and a great amount of manpower and resources are spent in keeping them at bay.

At Air Headquarter (HQ) in Delhi, one langur (the larger black-faced variety) is employed to scare away its smaller rhesus cousins. Its handler keeps it on a long leash to ensure that it doesn't escape. He comes with the langur perched on the rear seat of his bicycle. However, at Gorakhpur, the two cousins have developed an astonishing comfort zone. Along the main road in the residential complex, one side each is dominated by the two in complete harmony, much to the utter consternation of the residents. In their playfulness, they damage water tanks, pipes, fittings and, of course, pick up anything edible within their reach. Everything has been tried—crackers, sonic guns, and what have you, but to no avail. Such is the power of Bajrang Bali.

## Annoying Antelope

Airbases all over are great havens for wildlife, including a variety of birds, antelope, porcupines and jackals. The list goes on. These areas are relatively undisturbed by humans, and animals have learnt to live with the sound of jet engines. However, large animals such as deer and nilgai can pose great danger to aircraft taking off, especially at night. A pilot is blind except where his light is focused, and an animal is blinded and transfixed by the same light. Nilgai, or blue bulls, wrongly termed so since they are antelope, are docile but very strong. While chasing one in Sarsawa on a motorcycle, I saw a nilgai take a leap over a ten-foot barbed wire fence to escape. It did not manage to clear it, but it took the whole fence and a couple of cement pillars along with it.

But the best display of strength I saw was on one early winter morning when my squadron-mate Delta was driving to work in his brand-new Maruti-800. His horn startled a female nilgai, which took a leap and crash-landed on his bonnet. She got up, shrugged and ran off. But Delta's car was a mess, with the bonnet and some of its interior completely crushed. At bases like Tambaram in Chennai, the airfield is swamped with spotted deer or chital. However, they have some traditional paths where they cross the two runways. Thanks to adequate manpower deployed at night, there has never been a report of a deer-and-aircraft collision. At Allahabad, now called Prayagraj, an enclosure has been made for a deer park, which was inaugurated by former chief minister Vijay Bahuguna in the 1970s. It boasts of almost a hundred blackbucks, a highly endangered species. Despite repeated offers to the wildlife department, there have been no takers for relocating them. They believe the enclosure at the airfield is the safest for them. Certainly a dilemma for an airbase.

# AISA BHI HOTA HAI

THIS TITLE LITERALLY means 'this too can happen'. For many decades in India, civil helicopter companies were in minuscule numbers. Therefore, air force helicopters ended up serving all state governments and other agencies in every conceivable task and role. Some of the following stories bring out the unbelievable convergence of chance, luck, the uncanny, the supernatural and religion, and many other ingredients that always spring surprises.

From rescuing a kidnapped schoolboy in Shillong to the ordeal of a young widow after a helicopter crash in Car Nicobar Island, from a missing (later found) air warrior in Leh to a unique survival tale of pilots in the Lushai Hills of Meghalaya—the stories here cover this and much more.

## Kidnap Kahani

This might seem like an unbelievable tale, but what I recount is absolutely true. It happened in 1983 in India's Northeast. I was newly posted as a pilot officer to my squadron, the Himalayan Dragons. This rank has since disappeared because officers are now commissioned straight as flying officers. I was on a detachment to Guwahati airbase as a co-pilot to squadron leader Kishore of the local communication squadron. We flew a Chetak helicopter and the job was mainly milk runs to and from Shillong, where the command headquarters is located. It is a hill station at an altitude of almost 6,000 feet. The advance landing ground, or ALG, was made of vintage steel perforated sheets, with very rudimentary services for helicopter operation. Today, of course, Shillong ALG is a modern state-of-the-art complex. We did these milk runs almost every day and sometimes multiple ones. However, rarely were we tasked with flying beyond 3 p.m. since weather normally deteriorated by then. Also, no movement of senior officers took place beyond that time.

One weekend in August 1983, we had almost packed up for the day when we were ordered to fly immediately to Shillong. Moving as fast as possible, we managed to land there by 3 p.m. An air commodore briefed Kishore on the situation. It turned out that the child of an air force sergeant had gone missing from the school within the IAF area. It was quite likely that he had been picked up on the main road as witnessed by some children. This had happened before noon, and since then, a massive search operation had been launched by local police and IAF personnel. There was disquiet among the families, and it was therefore decided to rope in a helicopter survey too. And that's how we came in. However, it was like finding a needle in a haystack. We were told to circle all over Shillong, especially over the IAF cantonment. We did that for two hours and then had to land back at Guwahati because of sunset. The next day, we were ready and waiting for the weather conditions to clear in Shillong. Kishore briefed me on 'no joy' on finding the kid, and that we were required to continue circling Shillong with the assumption that the child was somewhere there. We reached the ALG, circled around for the next hour and landed back.

Despite our protests, we were asked to do the same after we had refuelled. Now Kishore decided to humour me a little. He asked me if there was anything I wanted to do or see. Recalling my geography lessons at school, I knew that Cherrapunji, once listed as the rainiest place on earth, was not too far away. I suggested a quick overfly so that I could boast about it to people back home. Once airborne, we circled around the IAF area and Shillong for half an hour before Kishore set course for Cherrapunji. We were there in fifteen or twenty minutes and he handed over the controls to me saying, 'Do what you want to for the next five minutes.' The rice basin below was beautiful and I flew around without a care. At this, Kishore, an ex-fighter pilot, taunted me to be a little aggressive. I took the hint, picked up a single Khasi hut away from the main road and started doing low dummy dives on it. After a few such antics, Kishore took over to head back. After landing, we were told to go back. The mood all over was sombre and morose.

That night at Guwahati, while I was in the bar washing a few down with my transport coursemates, I received a message from Kishore to report to the unit early. The next morning, he seemed worried because of a call the previous night from Shillong to 'get to the ALG fast'. We were there by nine because of the weather again. There was a huge crowd of IAF officers and men gathered, and the only hint was smiles and handshakes all around. Senior officers welcomed us and Kishore was singled out for praise.

The story was that the local police had found the boy by the main road in Cherrapunji late in the evening. The kidnappers had temporarily holed up in, believe it or not, the same hut that we had mock-attacked! After we had gone, and assuming they had been discovered, they untied the boy and fled. Local Khasi villagers around Shillong then told IAF personnel about certain secluded sects that believed in child sacrifice before putting in the foundation stone of a house. It was plain luck ordained from someone above—or maybe just a geography lesson in school!

## Close Shaves

Flying is inherently risky, especially military helicopter operations that demand virtually every conceivable trick in the book to be put into play. It is one of the reasons chopper guys are compulsive and intuitive improvisers. So, let me go down memory lane to share some risky incidents and jugaad efforts. There are stories among pilots about those who have trouble trailing them forever. Scientists have tried to explore the link between innate motor skills, situational awareness and the propensity to be involved in incidents and accidents. There is nothing conclusive as yet. But let me relate four instances where providence had definitely something to do with my being alive today. Lady Luck truly has a bigger role to play in how events unfold than most of us credit her with.

### Hara-Kiri

In the summer of 1989, I was posted to the Flying Dolphins in Car Nicobar in the Andaman Sea. I was flying an air test as a captain with a very senior wing commander as co-pilot. Lohtia was a very experienced Mi-8 pilot but had been posted as a chief operations officer, which involved very little actual flying. Biswas, the flight engineer and a core member in the cockpit, was also very experienced, with almost 5,000 hours under his belt. In fact, I was the least experienced among the crew but had signed as captain.

The Mi-8 was an old workhorse and barely able to sustain operational status. So air tests were important to categorize helicopters for long-duration sorties over the Indian Ocean. I was busy with my test profile in the air. Inexplicably, Lohtia decided to liven things up by wanting to switch off the engine that was running idle in the test profile. It would normally not have made much of a difference since the other engine was running on full power. However, without saying anything, he tapped Biswas and mistakenly gestured with his finger 'one back'. But 'one' was the live engine! Biswas asked, 'Confirm one?' Lohtia put a finger on his lips to quieten him and nodded. Without further ado, Biswas turned off the live engine.

I was oblivious to all this, concentrating on my turn to get down on to the runway, when suddenly we fell like a stone from the sky, from a height of 200 feet. Instinctively, I pushed the control stick fully forward and managed to gain some speed. The rotors of the chopper slowed to 70 per cent, a figure that no sane Mi-8 pilot will believe happened or is possible. There was barely any perceptible control left in my hands. To cut a long story short (though it may have taken only a few seconds), I pulled the control stick into my stomach for a semblance of a flare. We escaped hitting coconut trees, banged and bounced on the runway six times, and finally stopped. For many years, people did all kinds of calculations to figure out how we managed this—but there are no answers yet. Anything could have happened, including the slowed-down rotors cutting off the tail boom catastrophically. Lohtia, who had set out to surprise me, was in shock and awe for the rest of his tenure—he never flew again!

## Satya and Jape

In the same unit at Car Nicobar, another providential escape happened in the last month of my stay there. I was to fly a courier for the navy between the islands of Kamorta and Great Nicobar. It was going to be a long day so I wanted to start early, not later than 8 a.m. My Mi-8 helicopter was ready, all tanked up with twenty-two life jackets for the courier passengers. These jackets inflate automatically when in water. I had almost reached the helicopter when an airman ran up to me to say that the flight commander wanted to speak to me.

Since the Aircrew Examining Board was coming the next week for categorization, two pilots who were appearing for upgradation, Satya and Paranjape, wanted to do an exam profile that would take an hour and a half. I did protest initially but agreed later, since Satya was a good friend and Jape was a coursemate. They were airborne for a local overhead sortie and were in radio contact with the base for ten minutes. After that, there was total silence. After about half an hour, when innumerable calls were not responded to, emergency recovery was sounded.

Two more Mi-8s got airborne with many pairs of eyes on board. We divided the probable areas and systematically searched for the next two hours, but to no avail. There was not enough time and light to do an aerial search any more that day, so the focus shifted to other issues. Jape was staying alone while Satya's wife was carrying—they had got married about a year ago. The next day, a naval armada of seven ships that was exercising near Hut Bay joined in the search. Despite a week's search, nothing was found. We had also started a ground search in the island's dense tropical forest along with about 150 Indian Army soldiers especially flown in. The aerial search expanded geographically though it was highly improbable that they would have gone far. Nothing was ever found—not even the twenty-two self-inflatable life jackets that are bright orange to attract attention.

The story now takes a strange and even more unfortunate turn. Satya's parents and relatives reached the island on the third day and stayed on for almost a month. The search kept getting prolonged at their insistence. The father even made a trip to Port Blair to see a certain Muslim holy seer. He made a child look into a slate—on which children write with chalk—and gaze into the future. He predicted that all of them were safe on an island and would be found after seven years! It was ensured that Satya's wife, so vulnerable in grief and pregnant, got to know of this. The CO and all of us in the unit tried to reason and trash this superstitious rubbish, but the mental damage was done. Many years later, my wife met the good lady in Noida (near Delhi). She had never remarried and was bringing up a lovely daughter. Everything was normal, except that she still firmly believed that Satya would return.

### Deepak's Flicker

The third close shave I had was at Air Force Academy, where I was a flying instructor on IAF trainers such as Kirans and Deepaks (HPT-32). I had just returned from a sortie and handed over a 'running' HPT-32 to a cadet for his sector solo. Ensuring everything was normal, and since the cadet was confident, I gave him a thumbs up and went away. After about half an hour in the air, the cadet found his windshield completely covered with black oil and the cockpit full of smoke—he could see nothing outside. Seeing the imminent danger, the control tower ordered him to bail out from a fairly low height. It was the first successful bailout from this aircraft, and he showed great presence of mind and mental agility in executing it.

### Jaan Bachao (Save Yourself)

My next real-life incident was truly a life-or-death situation. I was posted at Shillong as Eastern Air Command's (EAC) controller of all helicopter operations. Air Marshal 'Raja' Goel was the senior air staff officer, or SASO, and in light of certain incidents, had called for a meeting of major functionaries at Guwahati. I was to accompany him in a Chetak helicopter from Shillong around 7.30 a.m. At the ALG, the captain (Gangs) briefed Raja on a thunderstorm midway, which might require a little diversion. Raja occupied the third seat in front as a passenger with headsets to communicate with the two pilots. I sat behind without any headset but with my seatbelts on.

All was good till we approached the cumulonimbus (technical name for a dangerous cloud that holds a thunderstorm). Some conversation took place among Raja and Gangs on the intercom; I saw him give a thumbs up to the captain. Now the chopper started going lower below the dark clouds, entering a valley. It started drizzling and then came a bolt from the blue. I felt the lightning was right next to us. It started pouring and visibility dropped as Gangs too dropped his speed. In spite of being an older, or even a bolder, chopper pilot, even I had panicked by now and started looking for landing fields in the barely discernible valley bottom.

Before going further with the story, let me explain what disorientation in pilots is. It has always been the greatest threat to chopper pilots since the machine, despite being fully flyable, has an 'unserviceable' pilot. In a nutshell, a pilot gets a feel of something happening despite the instruments showing otherwise, in the absence or impairment of visual cues. In the darkness and pouring rain, it happened to Gangs. His co-pilot was a recently commissioned flying officer, Tiwari, who was blissfully unaware of the impending danger.

Suddenly, while I was still looking for a forced landing field, the chopper entered the dark clouds above, and when my eyes instinctively went to the instruments in front, Gangs had inadvertently put on ninety-degree bank and power was on maximum (both way beyond limits). All was over I thought, and it must have taken me a fraction of a second to respond, but at that time, it seemed like an eternity. I yelled the choicest of expletives at Tiwari to take over controls, at the same time cursing Gangs to let go. After some kicking, pawing and yelling from behind, it finally happened. I now started shouting recovery actions to Tiwari like 'dump collective', 'stick to the left'—as if I was flying the chopper. Thankfully, he followed my 'colourful' orders exactly. We came tearing out of the clouds and narrowly skimmed the mountain sides before I could guide him to the fields below. It was still pouring, but I could discern an opening ahead that would lead us to Guwahati. I yelled to Tiwari to go that way.

We finally reached Guwahati—drenched in sweat rather than rain. Raja refused to go back in the Chetak after the meeting and asked for a bigger and safer Mi-8 helicopter. Back at the HQ the next day, Raja divulged only two things to everyone. First, in all his 12,000 hours of flying, he had never come this close to death. And second, he thought he had the most colourful repertoire of Punjabi expletives but was proven wrong on that day. I remember only one thing—in the panic, I forgot that it was the seatbelts that were holding me back. Otherwise, I would have climbed over Tiwari and taken over the controls. I met Tiwari many years later. He too remembered the incident and reminded me of the kicks, nudges and language that he had got from behind.

There are many more personal stories of high risks taken in war and combat, but these four have a great deal to do with kismet or fate, and therefore, their inclusion. There is a Hindi adage, '*Dane dane pe likha hai khanewale ka naam*', meaning each grain of food is ordained to reach a certain mouth! I think one can also say that every air mishap is meant for a certain name—just joking!

## Fighting to Survive

This is another believe-it-or-not story about choppers from the Northeast. Our squadron in Hashimara did a year-round detachment of two helicopters at Aizawl in Mizoram. Flying was intense and covered the entire Northeast. Therefore, there were frequent trips from the mother base at Hashi to Aizawl, via Shillong, to replace helicopters. On one such trip, the captain was KK, there was co-pilot Doggy (yes, that was Dogra's nickname) and Guru, who was missing his girlfriend in Aizawl, as a passenger. It was September 1984 and incessant monsoon rains had just recently calmed down. It was Friday and the crew had planned to be back in Hashi by the next day. All was normal till the refuelling halt at Shillong ALG.

The weather towards Aizawl and Kumbhirgram, an alternate base for diversion, started deteriorating fast. Any pilot who has flown in the Northeast will readily agree that the biggest and most unpredictable challenge is the weather. Some male pilots refer to both the weather and aircraft as 'she'—alluding perhaps to their purported fickle-mindedness and unpredictability. Well, female pilots give it back by invoking 'he' for both! I suspect that the urgency of getting back the next day, as also Guru's 'love quest' for his girlfriend, affected the decision to make a try. Try they did—getting into deeper bad weather, till finally a point came where KK's skills kicked in and he managed to land the helicopter without any damage deep in a ravine. It was so heavily forested that it seemed like a miraculous feat. After landing, they kept calling on the radio but to no avail since the hills had boxed them in. Those were times when only one civil flight flew over the area in a day, and that had done so in the morning.

Overdue actions were thwarted by bad weather over the Khasi Hills for the next two days. The survival ordeal had just begun. There were no rations on board and just one bottle of water. The three pilots huddled through the night in the small chopper because the outside was full of crawling creatures of every variety. It rained intermittently, making things worse as the cabin had big leaks in many places. They conserved the battery, which had now become weak. The next day, they continued trying to make radio calls till the battery suddenly died out. KK and Doggy foraged around for some food but could not trust their judgement on the funny-looking coloured fruits and berries. They avoided them. Another long night was spent in a similar fashion, with the addition of some fearsome animal calls and grunts.

Meanwhile, back at the unit and EAC, all stations were on alert but deep down, people feared the worst since no contact had been established. By the second night, the CO was told to prepare for all eventualities. The third day was also dominated by bad weather and 'no joy' on radio efforts by many aeroplanes, including the only Indian Airlines flight. By evening, the CO asked me, as the adjutant, to prepare coffins and other actions associated with the worst possible eventuality. It was depressing and I could not put my heart into it—praying and hoping all the time.

By now, all three survivors, who had still not done their official survival course that IAF pilots undergo, had managed to eat some roots, banana shoots and a karela or bitter gourd-like vegetable. They were covered with leeches and all had loose motions. Fortunately, a trickle of fresh water, hopefully safe, was found and the rain helped. Guru was desperate and, in frustration, made one last radio call with the battery that lasted only a minute after being put on. Miraculously, this went through to an Indian Airlines Fokker Friendship aeroplane landing faraway at Agartala. After sometime, these coordinates were passed on to the IAF. It was party time again. The AOC ordered that the bar should be open the next afternoon for a celebratory session once the pilots were picked up. But the youngsters had already started rejoicing.

The next day, weather permitted a rescue only around 11 a.m. There was another cycle of disappointment as nothing was found at and around the reported site. The beer session was cancelled in Hashi. The coordinates were rechecked from the Indian Airlines office in Calcutta (now Kolkata). They were finally found around 3 p.m. and rescued. It took another two days to recover the helicopter with a fresh battery and fuel. Hashi was relieved, but celebrations were muted because of the see-saw unfolding of events that left everyone feeling drained. We all learnt our lessons, including me, on what to do in case of the death of air warriors. KK hated even looking at bitter gourds for a long time. Guru decided to give his heart to someone else who lived in a more accessible location. Doggy was too young, being just posted in, to learn any lessons. He continued being gung-ho about life and flying.

## Megh-Malhar

An almost repeat performance took place a year later. A new captain in the unit had just been cleared by the CO, Bertie. Sandy was an ex-Jaguar pilot who had moved to helicopters. I was detailed as a co-pilot to him during a trip to Paro in Bhutan. He was my senior, but I was far more experienced in the area and on helicopters. At Paro, we got a hint that the weather had deteriorated in and around Hashi. As captain, Sandy insisted that he would jot down the weather. I was a little worried since it was his wedding anniversary and the pressure to get back was obvious. In fact, one of the reasons for him to come on that day was to pick up some wine and whisky. He penned down the actual weather at the control tower and came down to discuss it with me. Visibility at Hashi was 2,000 metres and likely to hold for the next hour—so it was still good.

We took off and started getting into trouble the moment we came to the foothills. We were now at treetop height with no possibility of going back since the valley mouth was closed. Low clouds were drifting at our height and it had become ominously dark. Finally, I took over the controls after Sandy's initial reluctance to give them up. There was no place to land in the heavily wooded area, but then I saw a small tea garden and the compulsory small field used as a football ground—thanks to the Bengalis' love for the game. We just made it because while switching off, the downpour started. It lasted for an hour and there was no way to contact Hashi because the only telephone was not working. We did give some blind calls on our radio set but knew that it was out of range.

It was quite an ordeal to keep the villagers from touching and exploring this 'gift from the gods'. By now, we were completely drenched since we could not leave our chopper unattended. In the meantime, overdue action had started at Hashi. A convoy of crash fire tenders, recovery vans and other paraphernalia had started on the only and poorly maintained road to the valley mouth. Bad weather prevented any other aircraft or helicopter from helping. After about four hours, it cleared a little and we took off. Almost immediately, we were in radio contact with the control tower. The relief in the controller's voice was perceptible. Then came the inevitable request—intercept the convoy to make them head back. We followed the road and, almost halfway to Hashi, flew over them and confirmed that they were turning back.

We were both grounded for the inquiry that followed because the reported weather was actually 200 metres instead of the extra zero that we had put down. It finally came down to Sandy admitting to his error in taking it down in writing at Paro. I am sure that the anniversary party that evening at his house had something to do with the mysterious extra zero.

## Camp Vignettes

### Mighty Moustaches

Back in the mid-1980s, Jaisalmer's star attractions were the majestic fort that seems to hang in the sky and the dunes of Sam. But a lesser-known star in the tourist circuit was Karna Ram Bheel. His name figured in the *Guinness Book of Records* as the man with the longest moustache in the world. He would 'unfurl' them for the right amount. He was probably the most photographed inhabitant of Jaisalmer. Every evening, he would come to rest in a makeshift hut next to our guardroom, since he was not permitted to stay inside. He claimed that dacoits were seeking revenge and his head. Stories abounded about him being a dacoit till he found an easier and more rewarding employment. He was the one who told me why turbans got larger as you moved west, into tougher desert terrain towards Pakistan—because the rare water wells got deeper; implying that the turbans served as ropes to draw water with. In the late 1980s, news came that his headless body was found near the airbase. The story goes that his head was carried back to Pakistan by his brothers-in-law from his first marriage across the border.

## Domestic Helps

I am now going to pen down memories of some of the people who took care of my family and me in the last three decades. It provides a snapshot of the social fabric that is as important as the air force blue fabric. My first orderly in Hashi was Ganesh, a Gurkha casual worker. He worked for a few officers and we paid him on a monthly basis. Trust and faith were high; and in hindsight, he garnered more sympathy because he had a club foot. During my entire stay, I did not feel anything amiss, but then we hardly had any assets of value back then. Most of the money was frittered away—just like any youngster today.

There had been a few cases of mobike and scooter thefts that were never solved. Also, they were too few and far between to become a big issue. Except, I suppose, for the concerned owner. I was just posted out to Jaisalmer. One large An-12 was scheduled the next day for a fighter squadron detachment that was, luckily, headed to Jaisalmer. I made Ganesh pack my trunk and planned to send it along with my bike. The agreement with the fighter squadron was that they would use it in the detachment. My coursemate, Mair, who has passed away, had the onus of taking care of this. That night we had a bachelor's binge and I came to my room late after having one too many. My Yezdi mobike was standing in the corridor, safely locked with a padlock. To a bachelor, a bike was the most precious thing—even more than a girlfriend. Somehow, even in a drunken stupor and despite feeling very, very sleepy, I managed to think about my bike and instinctively groped for the keys on the stool next to the bed. The bunch wasn't there. I looked around, but to no avail. Remembering that I had to dispatch 'her' the next day, I frantically searched for the keys. Now a little more sober, I saw the bunch of keys next to the outer room window, with the window latch open. It was all done discreetly with the aim of recovering the keys from the outside and stealing the bike when everyone was asleep. I was never more sober than at that point of time.

The next morning, I managed to dispatch my stuff in time. On getting back, I confronted Ganesh. Initially, he feigned ignorance, but later confessed. He even admitted to stealing my music system, which I had assumed he had packed. Unfortunately, his sob story of dire financial straits prevented me from taking the right action. However, I did mention it to another officer before leaving Hashi. Sure enough, a few months after I left, Ganesh was grilled by the police in connection with another scooter theft case. He confessed to being the main guy behind a gang that operated just outside the base. So much for being gullible bachelors.

My next memory is of Kamra Ram in Jaisalmer. He was the opposite—unskilled but scrupulously honest. I got married in April 1986 and my wife joined me in our temporary quarters in this field posting. Kamra was a simpleton whose loyalty and honesty could be taken for granted, but the same could not be said for his application of mind. Once, when he was taking an inordinate amount of time in cleaning utensils in the kitchen sink, my wife went to check. With a metal scrubber, Kamra had half-cleaned out a non-stick pan! These pans were new and of great value then. But we were very fond of him. When I visited again seven years later, as part of the examining board, I was pleasantly surprised to find him enrolled permanently in the IAF.

Then there was Pehelwan in Sarsawa. He was as strong as a bull and the champion wrestler of the village close by. His main job was to get milk from the village and distribute it among the officers' houses. But he would also be ready to do all kinds of errands. I remember once when we were shifting houses, we asked for his help. My wife's eyes opened wide when she saw him carrying our 165-litre refrigerator on his back single-handedly! He was also the eyes and ears of the station for miles around. I met him after almost fifteen years as a much more plump and prosperous milk businessman who now owned a dairy. His handshake was as firm, strong and painful as earlier.

## Viru's Story

This is a tale from Leh, when I was commanding the high-altitude base. It is probably the toughest place as a posting, second only to Thoise across Khardung La Pass. Civilians who work here are mostly Ladakhis or from Kargil. But there are some from the mainland too—from as far as Bihar, Bengal and Uttarakhand. Facing virtually unliveable conditions, these boys brave it out in the hope of joining the IAF as a non-combatant (NC[E]) or a civilian. Most make it after seven to eight years of rigour if age is on their side. Unlike other places in India, they are locked in since air travel is too costly and a road journey takes ten days to just clear the mountains. Their fear of losing the job and its attendant opportunity makes their presence in Leh an imperative. Even if one wanted to help them, there was little anyone could do.

One such boy was Viru from Chamoli in Uttarakhand. He had lost his father early in life and had a mother and four sisters to support. Every six months, during the recruitment drive, he was the most motivated individual. He virtually stood first in all the tests, both physical and mental. Yet, he would unfailingly miss out due to being underweight or anaemic, or something else. My wife and I developed empathy for him, especially considering that he was the fittest of them all. We worked on him for a year, made him gain some weight and ensured that he fit the bill. He cleared the recruitment, standing first on merit. But before he could leave for Delhi to get enrolled, I moved on a posting to Lucknow, happy in the knowledge that we had helped a needy soul and got the IAF a truly fit non-combatant. Three years passed and we were in Allahabad now. One day, my wife received a call on her mobile. It was Viru, who almost immediately broke down into uncontrollable sobs.

The story went thus. On reaching Delhi, after almost all procedures had been completed, he was rejected on some vague and frivolous grounds. He was so dejected and depressed that he went back to Uttarakhand and started working as a helper at a roadside tea shop. A year later, that shop closed down and he was out of a job. Since then, he had been working as a labourer under the Mahatma Gandhi National Rural Employment Guarantee Act (MGNREGA), a government daily labour scheme. His spirit and will were completely broken. Then, as God generally wills it, a friend from Leh met him by pure chance. To cut a long story short, the friend knew about our soft corner for the boy. With great difficulty, he traced my wife's mobile number and forced him to call her. After some cajoling and speaking to his mother, we managed to get him to Allahabad. After a year's training, he once again made it because, thankfully, age was on his side. He joined the IAF as an NC(E), became the number one cross-country runner for Southern Air Command and now represents the IAF. What a turnaround!

### Rustom and Ismail

Another heart-rending story is of two Muslim brothers from faraway Bhagalpur in Bihar. The family was extremely poor and surviving on a hand-to-mouth existence with three girls and two sons. And then, with an utterance of 'triple talaq', the father left the family for another younger woman, never to be seen again. In dire straits, the mother approached her elder brother in Noida for help. He was not doing too well himself, but accommodated the six of them. However, to make ends meet, he handed (sold) the two small boys, aged seven and ten, to a hotel owner. For the next three years, the boys went through a harrowing experience of exploitation and slavery. Rustom, the elder one, took whatever care he could of his younger sibling, Ismail—one can still make out the difference in their physiques due to relative malnutrition. At the end of a gruelling three years, a chance encounter with an NGO working on child labour issues convinced Rustom to run away. The NGO helped by giving a dire warning to the hotel owner after the scooting. Rustom then joined his mother to help in every way to educate Ismail and run the house. He washed cars in the morning and did many chores for multiple houses along with his mother. He could neither read nor write, but made sure Ismail cleared his 10th standard board exams.

He used to clean our car and so, once in a while, I would greet him. One day, quite by chance, we got to know his story through our neighbour. It took us two years to train and guide Ismail to be recruited into uniformed services; however, his heart was set on joining the IAF. Even after joining as an NC(E), his commitment to his family and nation was remarkable. Within two years, he was commended by the Air Chief for his work during the Kashmir floods of 2014.

## Whimsical Waters

As a three-year-old child, I almost drowned in my village pond. I was an extra-curious brat, who had to do what everyone forbade. One of these never-to-do things was to go towards the local pond close to my maternal grandfather's house in a village next to the Ganges. It was a lazy afternoon when most menfolk were out at work and the women were inside the house resting or catching up on gossip. I managed to slip out to explore as only a child can. And then nature called. The nearest field was good enough, but it was the need to wash that almost cooked my goose. I went towards the slippery bank and, before I knew it, I fell in. I do not really remember anything clearly after that. What happened was that a local charwaha (cattle-herder) resting on a tree opposite saw my little hands thrashing around in the water. He rushed and held out his stick, which I somehow grabbed and was pulled out. Being the darling of my grandfather as a first child, the whole family was tense as they waited for him to arrive home in the evening. Fortunately, he was so relieved and thankful that I was alive, he actually forgot to blame or scold anyone.

Yet, I do not remember being scared of water while extensively swimming in rivers or oceans, or doing all kinds of adventures over or under water. Even an encounter with a whirlpool in the Siang river, which sucked me in for a full ten seconds despite my lifejacket, never deterred my love for nature, especially mountains and rivers. As cadets at the National Defence Academy (NDA), we had gone on a field trip to Mumbai. In the evening, our entire batch went to a beach called Silver Sand. While frolicking around, John, who later died at Air Force Academy in a crash, suddenly found one colleague trying to grab his legs. He held him by his hair and pulled him up. To his horror, it was the dead body of a teen in rigor mortis. We dragged the body to the beach. Another body surfaced after five minutes. It was then that a caretaker came up and told us that five school students had gone missing in the morning during a large school event. Three were still missing. That is the danger of unseen undercurrents that drown so many happy picnickers. We have had so many cases of officers or their family members drowning. I remember Mamgain, his son and brother-in-law—all non-swimmers—drowning while trying to save his son in Goa. The two wives stood helplessly on the secluded beach where no lifeguard was available.

Sangam at Allahabad is an iconic symbol for Hindus. Come the Kumbh or Ardh Kumbh, a sea of humanity descends on the confluence of the three rivers, i.e., the Ganga, Yamuna and Saraswati (which is mythical). The administration at Sangam is very adept at handling this chaos in a well-orchestrated plan. This includes a tent city, toilets, waste management, water supply and overall hygiene—all on an unimaginable scale. Not a single case of drowning or other such mishaps generally take place, such is the tight monitoring. It is also a great tribute to the simple religious faith of the community at large that allows itself to be channelized so easily.

Even beyond auspicious occasions, Sangam is popular on the religious tourism circuit of the country. Thousands come to take a dip in the holy confluence every day. A sizeable number of expert boatmen with a variety of boats are always present to ferry pilgrims. How courageous and expert they are we came to know after a touch of tragedy.

Some ten airmen who had been freshly recruited into the IAF had come on attachment to the airbase at Allahabad. As is inevitable, a trip to Sangam was quietly planned on a Sunday morning. The whole lot were non-swimmers, and perhaps did not fully grasp the inherent dangers in certain spots. Finding a less-crowded bank, four of them ventured into the seemingly shallow river. A sudden steep drop caught the lead airman by surprise and he started drowning. In a tragic sequence, one by one, each of them got trapped as they tried to save each other. Seeing the last two drowning, a boatman and his helper quickly rowed over. One airman's hands were still above the water and he was pulled up. The helper then dived and pulled up one more unconscious fellow, who was then revived. By now, others had also joined the rescue but the two bodies could not be located. As is usual, these floated out the next day.

There is one truly strange case of drowning that remains forever etched in my mind. I was commanding the airbase at Leh in 2013. I was out of the base since mid-June, handling the Uttarakhand disaster, when a drowning incident was reported. Four airmen had gone to the Indus for a picnic. Two strayed out towards the river bank. After sometime, a Khalsa airman returned saying he could not find Jhajaria, who hailed from Rajasthan. A search involving the army, police, boats and locals over a week yielded no results. The Khalsa airman claimed that he had looked away for a few moments, and when he turned around, Jhajaria was gone. I got a call from Leh while I was at Dehradun. All I could do was tell John (my second-in-command) to liaise with all agencies. I also spoke to the Superintendent of Police (SP), Leh, who was a good friend. The inputs were confusing and ambiguous. I instructed John to not declare Jhajaria dead till a full investigation was done.

I joined back at Leh in the first week of August. Jhajaria's father was calling up every day, asking for the case to be closed, since the family was in emotional turmoil. Everyone on the chain of command and the Air HQ was pressurizing me to declare him dead. There was even a call from a secretary in Rashtrapati Bhavan and an MP who raised the issue in Parliament. This deepened my doubts even further. The Khalsa airman did not change his statement throughout. A final call came from my commander-in-chief, who held me in high esteem. He cautioned me that I might regret this since a lot of higher-ups had got involved. But somehow, things did not add up, and I stubbornly held on. The daily nagging calls from the father continued. And suddenly, sometime in October, Jhajaria, escorted by his father, reported to the IAF Police in Delhi. He was later dismissed from service. The entire effort was connived to gain benefits, and a change of identity had been planned down to the minutest detail. But for a doubtful and stubborn base commander, they may have had their way.

## Work and Worship

The IAF is truly pan-Indian in its recruitment and constituents. Unique blends of secularism, where religion and rituals are truly private matters, exist across all air force institutions. Every major festival is celebrated with gusto, with a deeper message of not only respecting each other's cultures but also enjoying and revelling in it. And therefore, Holi, Diwali, Christmas, Eid and other festivals are celebrated by all. Every major foundation-laying or events such as the commencement of a flying course in training set-ups is preceded by a puja that is inclusive of a pandit, a maulvi, a priest and a granthi. This is distinctly different from a 'to each his own' philosophy.

It is also quite normal to have a cluster of places of worship in one corner of a station, all housed next to each other. These sarv dharma sthals, or shrines of all faiths, ensure no polarizations in the rich and diverse social fabric. Many bases have ancient places of worship located quite deep inside, even in core secure and prohibited areas. Over the years, they have developed processes that allow huge public gatherings and worship on certain occasions. These are security nightmares; however, the flip side is it allows a strong public connect. Let me start with the rare 'Reclining Vishnu' temple at the

Air Force Academy, which attracts large congregations from both inside as well as outside the campus on certain festivals. Then there is the old Shiva Temple in Hindon. On Maha Shivaratri, thousands from villages (and now the extended city of Ghaziabad) are escorted in for a massive two-day congregation. Air Force Station, Agra, follows a similar procedure for the Balhara Temple dedicated to Lord Shiva, which is the presiding deity of nearby villagers. These places are preserved as they have been for centuries—complete with peacocks, other birds and sometimes deer too. A mosque stands at the Jammu airbase, right next to the runway. Bakshi-ka-Talab is an IAF airbase next to Lucknow. It has a famous Brahm Baba shrine complete with a legendary banyan tree right next to where fighter aeroplanes start their daily missions.

Leh airbase has an acute shortage of space, and so an igloo serves as a community place of worship. Its main wall is possibly unique in that it has frames depicting every religion that exists in the country. No one has a problem saying his private prayers in the igloo. I must also mention an ancient banyan tree in Mohanbari, very close to where the Mi-17 workhorses are parked. A station commander decided to chop the tree down to increase the operational area sometime in the late 1990s. Barely had a few branches been pruned that an accident took place involving a Mi-17 in the Arunachal hills. As if by a community consensus, the tree-cutting was stopped, and it has never resumed till date. Superstition or faith, whatever you call it, runs deep in everyone.

A sun temple at the airbase in Bihta, near Patna, takes the cake. It comes to life during the most auspicious Bihari festival of Chhath. People from all across Bihar descend on this temple and its pond for three days to do puja. The sea of humanity allows hardly any movement, and yet the glow of faith on all faces is truly remarkable. The IAF truly goes out of its way to help and facilitate the puja in every possible way.

Operating with the Indian Army, one comes across dozens of legendary shrines dedicated to gods and men alike. In the late 1980s, Om Prakash, an artillery soldier, was sent on a patrol to Malaun Post in the northern Siachen Glacier. Reportedly, he single-handedly beat back Pakistani soldiers but never returned. His body was never found, but troops had dreams about impending dangers on the glacier, which reinforced their faith in OP Baba, and temples were built in his name. Mission reports are regularly given to him before and after operations. As pilots, every detachment was started with prayers at his shrine. Every one serving in the glacier believes he accords protection against not only the enemy but also ensures warnings of impending dangers of an extremely hostile nature.

The story of Baba Harbhajan Singh—the hero of Nathu La Pass in Sikkim—is even stranger. He was an Indian Army soldier who died on duty while providing supplies to troops on the Line of Actual Control (LAC). It is a firm belief among those posted there that his body may have left the world, but his soul is still on active duty. He was accorded the status of saint by the Indian Army and, as the legend goes, he himself helped the army locate his body three days after his death. A shrine was built at his samadhi in the mountains. Baba warns the soldiers of any impending attack at least a few days in advance. During flag meetings between India and China, a chair is set aside for him. His mandir today has three rooms that are cleaned every morning—office, store room and living room. In the living room, every item of his is neatly preserved—bed, shoes, slippers, water bottle, ironed uniform and even an umbrella. He draws a major's salary every month and gets two months of leave every year to visit his home town by train.

During the staff course at Wellington in Tamil Nadu, air force and navy officers are taken for a forward area tour—my group's was to eastern Sikkim. The high point, literally and figuratively, was Nathu La Pass. On the way back, we stopped at Baba Harbhajan's shrine, more as a tribute to the Indian jawan. Some of the officers declined to get down—some because they were tired, some because they thought it was hogwash. An old Junior Commissioned Officer (JCO) approached with folded hands and requested them to at least step down from the bus, but they did not relent. We started our downhill journey to Gangtok by 2 p.m., expecting to reach in two to three hours. Within half an hour, our bus broke down and we were stuck at a high altitude in failing light with no one in sight.

The Indian Army's recovery team got into action and we finally reached Gangtok well past midnight. But not before we went through a harrowing experience of temperatures below zero, winds with a high chill factor and clothing not really suited for these conditions. Suddenly, everyone remembered the episode at the shrine. You can well imagine who was at the receiving end of our collective curses!

### Jai Jai Shiva Shankar

I was brought up in a fairly ambivalent religious environment. All pujas and festivals were celebrated but more with the purpose of getting together and having fun under one roof. My parents took the path of spirituality under the umbrella of Radha Soami Satsang Beas with very little emphasis on one particular god but a lot on the synthesis of all good teachings of the holy books. The IAF, as mentioned earlier, is very open about religion—to each his own—and revels in the diversity. But I have noticed that my devotion to Lord Shiva has grown over the years. I commanded Siachen Tigers whose logo has a majestic *trishul* against the backdrop of Mount Kailash. While commanding the Tactical Air Centre in Srinagar, my bedroom window opened to a beautiful view of Shankaracharya Temple. This has a huge Shiva lingam dating back to the ancient times. As the air officer commanding (AOC) at Leh, I was deputed to oversee the massive response to the Uttarakhand disaster in 2013.

We ended up rescuing and evacuating lakhs of people who had gone to pray at Lord Shiva's shrine in Kedarnath. It was a great window to serve God by being useful to humanity at large.

As mentioned earlier, a Shiva temple in Leh, on the banks of the Indus, was my favourite haunt. Many airmen (who were also Shiva bhakts) requested that we contribute and tidy up the temple. We did, but the only problem was that the owner was a local—a drunkard and a no-good fellow. His only demand was that the 'daan peti', or offering chest, be his sole property. He had his own lock on it. In return, he let us do whatever we wanted. We ensured that the chest had just enough money to look after his petty needs—the real chest was in our temple at the airbase.

# ACTION CHRONICLES

# A GLANCE AT CHOPPER OPERATIONS

THIS SECTION BRINGS out the travails, professionalism, test of character and sheer joy of pilots doing what they do best—operations in war and peace. The diversity of backgrounds, circumstances and, as always, the humour will amaze readers.

From evacuating pregnant women from hillsides in Mizoram to numerous flood-rescue missions, the sheer complexities that await a pilot are what these stories are about. On the other side, wartime anecdotes—for example, in Sri Lanka, against the Chinese in Arunachal in 1986–87 and combating the Maoists in India's Red Corridor—will open the reader's eyes to the agony, joy and humour in the line of duty. And yes, there are crazy, unbelievable tales too, such as the search for YSR's ill-fated helicopter crash. Remember, he was the serving chief minister of the erstwhile united Andhra Pradesh.

## Aizawl Amalgam

Flying in Mizoram mainly involved supporting counter-insurgency measures of the army and government forces, as well as aiding civilians in every possible way. This was a time when there were no civilian helicopters around, and therefore, whether it was a chief minister or a common person who needed medical attention, IAF helicopters were hailed as saviours and heroes by one and all. It also made it easy for bachelor pilots to befriend locals, especially girls!

An iconic figure in quashing the remnants of the rebellion by the Mizo National Front (MNF) was Major-General Tomar, or 'Yogi'. I still consider him a role model and perfect for the situation at hand. He was a widower and put in at least eighteen hours a day at work. Scrupulously honest and someone who walked the talk in every way, he was feared and held in awe by both the MNF and the army. He would fly five days in a week and do his ground and staff work by night. He would insist that young pilots like me attend all briefings and discussions. We didn't enjoy it much since we felt there were more lucrative things to do. However, only later did I realize that understanding the deeper aspects of operations helped us empathize with the soldiers and, at times, put our own lives on the line for them. As part of his emphasis on a 'moral' campaign, he truly cracked down on financial impropriety and womanizing. I distinctly remember a major of a jeep company who underwent a court martial for having a 'keep'. It did wonders in winning the local population over. Often, we would fly in reinforcements to a combat zone and also fly out surrendered militants. In one such sortie, we carried five MNF insurgents, all tied up behind. The one memory that never goes away is the terrible stink in the chopper all the way to Masimpur near Silchar. It took a mere forty minutes, but at that time it felt like eternity.

## Mutiny in Tripura

The year 1984 was remarkable because of Operation Blue Star in Amritsar and its ramifications across the country for years to come. Mizoram was no exception, with many Sikh battalions and officers deployed all over the Northeast. Immediately after Operation Blue Star in June, all precautions were taken, but the rumblings were palpable. A Sikh regiment battalion, which was moving out from near Agartala in Tripura and was waiting for its special train, suddenly revolted and took over the 'kot', or armoury. All hell broke loose—they took over the liquor store of the officers' mess and finished every drop available. All officers made a run for it since the soldiers had started firing at will, but mostly in the air. We were told to plan the earliest take-off from Aizawl with the general on board with a radio set.

We took off before sunrise and were over the helipad in about forty minutes. The radio communication clearly indicated that a light machine gun had been positioned to take 'good care of the general'. We kept orbiting at 5,000 feet since there were reports of potshots being aimed at us. Finally, due to low fuel, we headed to Agartala. Now, the most extraordinary thing happened. A south Indian, Captain Radhakrishnan of the supply corps, managed to reach there in his jeep with only a driver and no weapons. It was forenoon, the effects of the liquor were waning and 'hosh' had returned. After an initial roughing-up, and the knowledge that two fully armed convoys of troops were headed their way, the mutineers accepted the captain's intervention. Arms were laid down; the armed soldiers entered and took over; and the general was finally allowed to land. The rest is a long story about how the battalion with a glorious past was finally disbanded.

## Jaisalmer Jaunts

The period of 1986–87 was of strategic importance for India with a young prime minister, Rajiv Gandhi, and an equally dynamic army chief, General Sundarji. It is said that the general was way ahead of his time. So true, because his strategic reach, or overreach as some consider it, covered Operation Pawan in Sri Lanka, Operation Falcon in Arunachal Pradesh, which was a war-like deployment against the Chinese, and Operation Brasstacks against Pakistan. I had the opportunity to be a participant in operations Pawan and Brasstacks. Here are some recollections.

Posted at Jaisalmer in 1986, in an airborne forward air controller unit, we were in the thick of things. The likelihood of the balloon going up was very high, and there were many false alarms. And yet, despite eyeball-to-eyeball stares, there were neither any bullets fired nor any untoward incidents, except one. A colleague who was made in charge of a deployed mobile unit decided to visit them for morale-boosting. All went well for the first few days with only his driver and him in their Willys jeep. And then came the proverbial wrong turn—and they were lost. Entering a village, they started to make inquiries. The headman was very honest—they had just entered Pakistan, but where was the enmity? He offered them camel milk and they got talking. It may have been just half an hour, but it was enough for Pakistan Rangers to arrive on the scene once the information reached them. The long ordeal of over a week of questioning, flag meetings and counter-questioning once they came back requires a separate chapter!

Since the face-off was a long one, the units posted there went through a lot of hardships and were truly exhausted by the time normality returned. Customary get-togethers such as rum punches were held. Those were times when not all officers drank whisky—some still swore by rum varieties such as Sea Pirate and Old Monk. How can you name an alcoholic drink 'Old Monk'?

The tradition of our airmen was to take half a glass of water and slowly pour the rum on top. This was the toast to a unit's 'izzat'—first a half glass of rum to light the fire in your tummy, then water chasing it down to quench it. COs used to have their favourites go through this ordeal because, in all likelihood, those young officers had to be carried away after a number of such toasts.

Our flight commander ORP (yes, those were his real initials and nickname) was a good man but very emotional about issues—he was fond of gesticulating and using hand symbols to make his point. One evening's discussion at the crowded bar was on air combat survivability. In his typical fashion, ORP, an ex-fighter pilot, was all over the place with both his hands depicting hard turns and what have you. Abruptly, the combat and his voice stopped with both his arms high up in the air. We waited, assuming this was part of the suspense. But no! ORP's shoulder had just dislocated—it was completely out of the socket. Later, we came to know that this was a normal problem and only those who were watching panicked. ORP gently reassured us, calmly went about some complicated manoeuvring to set it right and said he would complete this particular story some other time!

## Dakota Down

Here is an account of a once-in-a-lifetime accident that I was witness to. Our unit in Jaisalmer was put up in a temporary place close to the runway and taxi track. It had retaining walls (protection against aerial attacks) all around, which served a secondary purpose of offering a great view with the famed Jaisalmer fort in the background. Quite often, we used to have our breakfast on field tables and chairs.

One sunny day, I got delayed because of some adjutant-related duties and was having breakfast, enjoying the view of runway operations. A civil Dakota had just lined up. It was a courier for an oil company that was on an exploration bid in the Thar Desert. As the Dakota rose, I couldn't help reminiscing about this great design of an aeroplane that had served the world so well. All of a sudden, the Dakota banked ninety degrees, fell on to the runway, cartwheeled a couple of times and finally crashed. As it burst into flames, I could see figures escaping from the rear main door. Within no time, thick black smoke started rising up. It came out later that all sixteen on board had escaped, including a drunk pilot!

Within minutes, a crash fire tender approached at breakneck speed but broke down before it could reach the aeroplane. A second, following closely behind, reached and started its foam throw, which overshot the burning wreckage. A sergeant came out, climbed up from the windscreen side and started adjusting it with a spanner. In the meantime, an officer who had reached the site in his jeep approached the driver of the fire tender and asked him to reverse so that the foam throw could reach the fire. While reversing, the sergeant, who was focused on his adjustments, fell down and broke his arm. To cut a long story short—all occupants survived miraculously without a scratch, the wreckage burnt itself out since no foam could reach it, and the only casualty was a ground personnel with a broken arm. Such is aviation!

## Sojourns in Sri Lanka

After Jaisalmer, a hard-field area where I started my family, we moved all the way across India, and an ocean named after it, to Car Nicobar in the Andamans. It was to be an idyllic break with quality family time. It was, except for some interesting interludes in Sri Lanka as a Mi-8 pilot who was part of the Indian Peacekeeping Force. If there was a high-intensity counter-insurgency operation to be experienced, it was here. The main opposition was a highly motivated, intelligent and crafty bunch—the Liberation Tigers of Tamil Elam or LTTE. Its leader, Prabhakaran, who was finally killed in 2009, still evokes fear and admiration for his adaptability and ruthlessness.

There were four main bases where IAF operations were concentrated—Jaffna or Palaly airport, Vavuniya, Trincomalee and Batticaloa. From these bases, thousands of IAF aeroplane sorties provided the link and support to India, with a hub-and-spoke model of helicopter support to hundreds of helipads at army outposts. Initially, the going was crazy. Sometimes, in the same day, you could end up doing sorties and supporting the Indian Army, the LTTE or even some other rival militant groups such as Eelam People's Revolutionary Liberation Front (EPRLF)or People's Liberation Organization of Tamil Eelam (PLOTE). The issue was so complex and dynamic that strategy and tactics changed and evolved throughout. Some memories, however, are vivid.

## Ambushed

Once, while Kama and I were flying a support mission from Vavuniya to a southern outpost, we heard some urgent operational calls on the radio. The action was taking place at a helipad close by, and we were almost over it. An army Ranjit (light machine gun-mounted helicopter) was getting down to take out some LTTE rebels who had attacked an army camp. Abruptly, there were panic calls as if the radio of the Ranjit had got jammed in transmitting mode. A burst from an AK-47 had hit the Ranjit. While little damage was done by most bullets, one slug had broken the Perspex, hit the control stick of the captain (Daman), taking out his thumb, and hit the jaw of the co-pilot, a Sikh officer whose name I do not remember. Almost a dozen of his teeth had been dislodged and he was gagging on them. It was a commendable effort by Daman to fly the helicopter without the thumb of his flying hand, pass urgent instructions to the gunner to save the co-pilot's life and, at the same time, head back to Vavuniya. It was not only a brave task but one that showed his great presence of mind in a calamitous situation. All this was broadcast to everyone flying, since the transmit switch had jammed due to the bullets.

There was a similar scene that I witnessed in June 1989, while overflying a place called Pankulam on the road north to Killinochchi. A Jat regiment battalion's convoy had been ambushed. The CO had taken nine bullets and many others were injured. From the top, we could see the battalion get its act together and the LTTE cadres making a getaway in the face of sustained fire. The attack helicopter had been called in, but by the time it arrived, the LTTE had simply vanished. We really felt helpless since we were not armed for that mission.

The forces that were more than a match for the LTTE in every way were the Special Forces, or the Paras. I operated with 1, 2 and 10 Para in various missions. The most remarkable thing about them was how small teams were secretly placed during evening or night by slithering or winching down from a helicopter in an area they had designated. For the next few days, they would go about their act, negating the advantages that the LTTE had over the usual large-scale army operations. We would pick them up from a different location after a few days. It was an honour to operate with the Special Forces. With them, one gets a drift of the meaning of 'junoon' or passion in its truest sense.

## Mortar Mani

The threat on ground was far more sinister and difficult to manage than the one in the air. A number of cases of infiltration, even by women and children who blew themselves up, ensured that base protection was treated with utmost seriousness. We had our weapons with us at all times. Vavuniya was especially vulnerable because of the geography and the extant situation. There were multiple tiers of defence, as in a fortification. Once, when threat levels were declared high, the tension was palpable all across the camp. Whether it was a mischievous act or genuinely out of fear, a Sri Lankan soldier fired a burst of his machine gun in the night. More sporadic fire burst out from different parts, and within minutes the whole camp was letting out tensions—and all in the air. An early Diwali followed in the middle of a dark night, with thousands of rounds being fired.

Because of the geography, the camp was particularly vulnerable to mortar fire, and therefore, special measures were taken to alleviate the threat such as active patrolling and intelligence gathering. One day, the army boss called for a meeting of all units. There was credible intelligence that the LTTE were planning to use mortars to hit our helicopters on ground. These had been zeroed-in on by them. A decision was taken to park them at different places when we came in for last landing. This went on for a few days till logistical challenges forced a return to the earlier practice.

However, the really amusing story is another related incident. The air force camp was right next to the runway. It was a square set-up around a large volleyball court with tents arranged all around, including the larger mess tent. The base commander (IAF) was Groupie Sahota, a fighter pilot whose tent was similar to everyone else's on the outside but better done up inside. He was of a very empathizing and decent disposition, but he was clearly out of his comfort zone. Ravi, the chief engineering officer, a witty and intelligent officer, was very fond of pulling Sahota's leg whenever an opportunity presented itself.

During the mortar high alert, when we had gathered for our usual drinks before dinner, he told us that the latest inputs and analysis had revealed that the LTTE believed getting helicopters and pilots was not worth it because they could be replaced. What was crucial was to get the leadership—to cut the head off. Sahota, too, was listening intently. Ravi went on to explain that, at night, any assassin would recognize our commander's tent by the unique white jeep parked in front of it, and therefore, it called for a dispersal plan just like the helicopters. Realizing the joke, all of us laughed; but in hindsight, Sahota's laughter seemed a little nervous.

We went to bed and, as usual, fell off to sleep instantly after a gruelling day. I used to share my tent with Atri, another pilot. He would get up ten minutes earlier, since he was junior to me, to ensure the staggered use of the common toilets. The next morning, before the sun rose, he got into his routine and went out of the tent. Instantly, he came back and woke me up, laughing loudly all the time. Lo and behold, the white jeep was parked in front of our tent, while our olive-green jeep was in front of the commander's. When confronted, Sahota assured us that it would be parked randomly every night. Ravi had struck—again!

## Suicide Bombing: Pioneers

The first mass suicide by seventeen LTTE prisoners by swallowing cyanide capsules took place in October 1987. This set the tone for what was to follow. Till then, terrorism was about brazen attacks—some even leading to martyrdom but never as a calibrated suicidal, tactical action. The Indian Army suffered quite heavily in the process, with even children and women being used as suicide bombers. One had to be really careful when going to markets. The only solution was randomness and not establishing a pattern or routine. But it was a pity that you had to look suspiciously at any child or lady approaching you. After the LTTE's experiments, suicide-based terrorism has grown exponentially. Today, it is the cheapest and most effective form of attack used by terrorists.

## Special Ops: Brothers in Arms

### Fear the Dragon?

The debacle of 1962 sits very heavily on the Indian psyche. Till quite recently, a Chinese soldier was imagined to be ten feet tall. Forgotten are the many episodes since then that have pricked this balloon or myth. Choppers had just about been inducted in the late 1950s, and therefore, were unprepared and unimaginatively employed by the Indian forces during the 1962 war. However, they did yeoman service in supporting the army's retreat, including casualty evacuation, supply drop and recce sorties, among others. Squadron Leader Saigal became the first chopper martyr when, while on a rescue sortie, his Bell helicopter was overrun by the Chinese forces. He was never heard of again. Mi-4s, barely inducted into the IAF, did hundreds of sorties in the most difficult circumstances, sometimes under fire. Whole battalions were inducted into strategic locations in Ladakh, right under China's nose.

It was in the 1965 war that choppers were gainfully employed to blunt the onslaught of the Pakistani Razakars. Hundreds of logistics missions were carried out to support our beleaguered army. However, it was the modification and use of the Mi-4 as an armed helicopter that clinched the issue and turned the tide against Pakistan's Operation Gibraltar. A gun of heavy calibre from a World War II Liberator bomber was retrofitted as a front gun. Railings were fabricated and fixed on the cargo compartment floor to hold and drop bombs from the rear with the help of deployable chutes. All the trials were done in Chandigarh in just over a week—followed by the modification of ten Mi-4s. Operating as a six-helicopter detachment, the Mi-4s did almost a hundred armed sorties, inflicting great damage to the positions and morale of the Razakars. They could quickly and as easily switch over to a supply role for our manoeuvring army across Jammu and Kashmir. General Harbaksh Singh, the then army commander, wrote highly about them.

Speaking of the fear of the dragon, 1967 was a watershed period across Nathu La. In belligerence, the People's Liberation Army (PLA) had transgressed to dominate Sikkim. The Indian Army gave a befitting riposte, killing hundreds of Chinese soldiers (there's a Bollywood movie being made about this gallant but forgotten action). Now, fast-forward to 1986. Tensions were building up across the Line of Actual Control (LAC) between the two countries. A PLA regiment pushed forward in the Tawang sector, making permanent structures and helipads in contested but so far peaceful no-man's land. Prime Minister Rajiv Gandhi showed resoluteness and allowed an Indian brigade to be deployed and sustained in Zimithang, leading to an eyeball-to-eyeball situation. This was done with the help of Mi-8s and the recently inducted and powerful Mi-17s. The crisis escalated with the forward movement of up to thirteen Chinese divisions. India countered this move by deploying three full divisions in Arunachal and having another seven ready to move in Assam's plains. The stand-off lasted almost a year and was admirably supported by the IAF's helicopter fleet. It was the only means of sustenance in the mountains. This Indian operation was aptly named Operation Falcon.

## Special Heli-Borne Operations (SHBO)

While helicopters as war machines, vital suppliers and gunships were first used in France's Algerian Campaign in the 1950s, it was the Vietnam War that brought them to the fore as a game-changer. Chopper employment was truly only limited by a commander's creativity and risk-taking limits. The whole world sat up and took notice—and so did some Indians, especially two who changed the course of the war for the liberation of East Pakistan in 1971. General Sagat Singh was a maverick of the Indian Army and not very well liked by peers and superiors. But he had seen what Mi-4s could do during the 1966 Mizo campaign by Indian joint forces. During the 1971 war, he commanded 4 Corps that was to launch a secondary attack from the east (Tripura). And into his hands fell the eleven Mi-4s of 110 Helicopter Unit (HU) in Kumbhirgram. He had in tandem an air task force commander, Group Captain Chandan Singh, a transport pilot who could match him as a risk-taker. Together, they did the unthinkable and produced a miracle that only the fog of war can throw up.

Using Mi-4s to launch whole battalions of Gurkhas across the innumerable waterways, deemed as impassable as the famed Maginot Line, the enemy was outwitted and put in a grave decision dilemma. Gen. Niazi took the fatal call to defend Sylhet town with his two potent brigades, leaving the bridges and access to Dacca open, though it was never an objective of the Indian game plan. Gen. Sagat's 4 Corps was sitting on the doorstep of Dacca. He was made to wait there for a week not by the Pakistani opposition but by higher-ups in the army chain of command. It was the single act that made Dacca fall finally. And Bangladesh was born. Kudos to the Mi-4s and their crews, the 110 HU and the indomitable Indian soldier.

Since then, SHBO (especially slithering) has been the preferred mode of both the Special Forces and the infantry brigades. I was fortunate to be part of this action many times in Sri Lanka (IPKF) and during the Kargil War of 1999. I have also, like hundreds of other chopper pilots, done this in J&K and the Northeast. The operation in Jammu sector at the end of the new millennium's first decade is a masterclass. It was called Operation Hill Kaka, named after a pivotal mountain infested with insurgent camps and part of the larger operation named Sarp Vinash. It was an exceedingly successful joint operation based on trust and mutual understanding. Ahead of the operations, after joint consultations, the army began to discreetly prepare three helipads at critical points. This was followed by a mix of ground-based and heli-borne assaults by the infantry and Special Forces. At the end, according to army estimates, almost a hundred key terrorists from across Pakistan lay dead.

## A Special Breed

Special Forces (SF) across the world possess unique levels of training, skill and motivation. I was very fortunate in my career as a chopper pilot to interact with SFs of all types. 'They are different' does not sum them up—'they are truly special' does. My first experience was in Sarsawa, in Mi-17s, at the abode of 1 Para—Nahan. My NDA coursemate Anand was part of it. While joking in the bar about the 'ethos of madness' of the SF, as I termed it, he almost killed me with a blow to the larynx. Thereafter, I always took the SF very seriously. Training for slithering, and other crazy insertion modes, demonstrated the creed of the commandos very clearly. My real combat experience was in Sri Lanka during the IPKF sojourn. Any major offensive had large doles of special operations to provide the crucial edge. In fact, SF actions were far more successful and effective than large campaigns. It was normal for us to drop a team in a far-off jungle site and pick them up from another place after two days. In the interim, they managed to do considerable damage to LTTE camps and cadres. They would carry lungis to look like the rebels. I think the LTTE cadre feared only two things—SF action and Mi-25 gunships. On call Mi-25 and Mi-8 action to support these Paras were the riskiest and also the most exciting missions.

In 1989–90, the training area of the National Security Guard (NSG) came up at Manesar near Gurgaon. My squadron was actively involved in cross-training with them and acting as advisers to upgrade facilities for helicopter-borne training. It was fun trying new methods and innovative solutions such as quick rooftop insertions. A memorable mission that was planned at the Eastern Air Command was a joint one against the United Liberation Front of Asom (ULFA) camps in Bhutan. With Bhutan's permission, a mix of SF SHBO and rocket attacks by Mi-17s on a large ULFA camp caught them with their guard down. In fact, this was the precursor to the now-famous 'surgical strikes' in Myanmar and then Pakistan Occupied Kashmir in 2017–18.

IAF's elite commando force is the Garuds. As a TAC commander in Srinagar in 2006–07, I used to coordinate joint missions of Garud with the SF. They were as good as any other—given a chance. Unfortunately, this was later stopped, robbing them of valuable actual action experience. It started again in 2017, and Garud rose to the challenge—a posthumous Ashok Chakra (the highest peacetime gallantry award) is testimony. The next action that I personally witnessed was during the 2013 Uttarakhand disaster. After the wreckage of one of our choppers was found on a cliff at almost 8,000 feet, the remains had to be guarded against wild animals. A team was winched down under the most difficult conditions and fading light to spend a lonely, cold and risk-filled night with the mortal remains of those in the chopper. The next day they participated in recovering the remains of twenty martyrs.

A singular quality of the SF that never ceases to amaze is their adaptability, and also their junoon.

### Choppers Save Lives

The one thing an IAF helicopter pilot has surely done is save lives—in more ways than are imaginable. There are so many stories to tell that it would require a few books to do so. I am going down memory lane to recount some that I was involved in or saw.

#### Jhoom–Jhoom

There is a peculiar agricultural tradition in Mizoram known as 'jhooming'. Mizo tribals set fire to entire hillsides to sow seeds, with the ash acting as a fertilizer. After very inefficiently sowing their crop and harvesting it, they move on to the next hillside. It may have been okay earlier with lesser population, but now it is a recipe for an ecological disaster. Be that as it may, the real problem for chopper pilots was the thick smoke that engulfed the Lushai Hills for months. You could see nothing ahead, especially at higher speed. Actual in-flight visibility often dropped to zero. Now, a Chetak is a very rudimentary seat-of-the-pants flying machine that is not cleared for cloud flying, or in abysmal conditions. These few months were really tough on us since the entire populace depended on IAF helicopters for emergency medical care.

I remember the case of a pregnant woman who had taken refuge under a tree during a thunderstorm on one such 'jhoomed' hillside. She had been struck by lightning and was critical. The chief medical officer at Aizawl, who knew us well, had not even projected an evacuation requirement, given the poor visibility. However, we got whiff of it from his assistant under the cover of anonymity. Finally, we took off in bad visibility with a clear mind that no untoward risk would be taken. We did manage to pick her up from the fields, where she lay for forty-eight hours with only her husband, since all the other villagers had gone home. Actually, the really difficult task was to put her in the helicopter since we could not fully land due to the slope. My co-pilot, Tawade, who has now passed away, unstrapped and helped, and we managed to get her to the hospital at Aizawl. Unfortunately, while she survived, the baby died. Hopefully, she went on to having other babies later.

## Sarsawa Serenade

On 13 October 1992, the hauling cable of a cable car carrying passengers to Timber Trail resort near Shimla in Himachal Pradesh had snapped. It was stuck with ten passengers in the middle of a valley. The IAF was requested to rescue them since the cable car was dangling at a height of 1,500 feet above the river bed and could collapse any time. As the rescue mission could not be undertaken after sunset, it was launched the next morning. An initial attempt was made by a smaller Chetak helicopter. It was found to be unsuitable because of the inadequate length of its winch cable and was replaced by a Mi-17 helicopter from my squadron—Mighty Armours. Paritosh Upadhyay, or Uppi, was tasked to undertake this hazardous mission because no other senior pilot was available. His co-pilot was the CO who had just converted to the Mi-17 and had little experience. The only solution was winching the passengers up from the cable car, for which the helicopter had to hover precariously close to the cables that ran above the cable car. The operation from the hovering helicopter had to be manoeuvred deftly in order to pick up people through a maze of twisted cables that were holding up the suspended cable car. It was fraught with danger—the slightest mistake by any team member could spell disaster.

Uppi manoeuvred to position himself above the cable car; the dimensions of the car's roof were approximately 2 ft × 2 ft. At that height, there was no visual reference for guidance for steady hovering and position-keeping. Turbulence and strong winds made precision hovering even more difficult and hazardous. To complicate matters, the winch of the Mi-17 helicopter had to be accurately passed through the narrow opening of the cable maze to lower Major Crasto of 1 Para on to the top of the suspended cable car. Five people were rescued in this manner till night set in and operations had to be stopped. The remaining five were rescued the next morning—imagine the night they had. Even under ideal conditions, hovering at heights is a tiring exercise and difficult to do over a long period. To do this under adverse conditions, for twenty minutes at a time for each of the ten survivors, involved exceptional courage, skill and team work. This rescue operation is perhaps the first of its kind in the world. Hats off, Uppi!

## Challenge at Chapakhowa

I was commanding a Mi-17 unit in the Northeast. It was December 2000. Below the calm and idyllic conditions of upper Assam, a battle was raging north of the Brahmaputra, in the densely forested foothills. ULFA militants were on the run, actively pursued by security forces of the unified command. On 13 December 2001, around 6.30 p.m., a patrol of the security forces was ambushed near Chapakhowa village, which lay north of the Brahmaputra, in the foothills of Arunachal Pradesh. Two soldiers were dead while four had multiple bullet injuries and were fighting to stay alive. With seven channels of the mighty Brahmaputra to be crossed by night to get to the nearest hospital, time was running out for the critically injured, who included an assistant commandant of the BSF, two constables of the Assam Police and one havildar of the Indian Army.

It was with this background that the mountain division at Dinjan approached me with a request for immediate casualty evacuation. I was officiating as station commander of Mohanbari base, and my first response to the request was that it would be done at first light. Around 8 p.m., the commander of the brigade concerned, a veteran NSG commando and winner of three gallantry medals, rang up saying that he was in radio contact with Chapakhowa. The medical officer on duty there had confirmed that three of the injured soldiers required immediate evacuation and at least two would not make it till first light. I advised him to get in touch with the Corps HQ to apprise senior officers at HQ EAC, Shillong, of the situation.

In the meantime, the helicopter was readied and the crew was decided. Though I did not expect to take off until first light, my flight commander, Atri, was tasked with planning the still improbable mission. The brigade let us know the details of obstructions around the only suitable landing field, a small ground surrounded by trees. In turn, I advised them to place the only vehicle available in one corner, which was to turn its headlights on when they heard the chopper. I had carried out a few missions by night during Operation Pawan and the Kargil War but never to an unprepared and unsurveyed site. Atri too had lots of experience in Sri Lanka and had over flown Chapakhowa by day a few times. He remembered that there was a huge wireless tower east of the village and the densely wooded area around. Another call to the army ensured that the soldiers would climb the tower with some sort of lights or torches to be flashed at us.

The mainstay of the mission was moonlit conditions with a full moon just three nights back. One additional flight gunner was arranged to be on board to ensure visual clearance on both sides and the rear. A conscious decision was made to make the approach into the moon, which would offer better visibility. This kind of mission had never been attempted in the area under the EAC and the army's Eastern Command; therefore, a delay was expected, if not a complete refusal. However, at 9 p.m., the call from HQ EAC came through. Air Marshal McMahon listened to my views, risk assessment and the pros and cons of the mission. The orders were simple—the blokes were required to live to fight another day; however, flight safety was paramount. In a gesture of tremendous faith and confidence in a field operator, they cleared me to do whatever I thought was the best course of action.

We took off within fifteen minutes of the 'go' call, in darkness under radar cover from Dinjan. Navigation to the point thirty-five minutes away was no problem with onboard GPS. Though a shallow fog had started engulfing the north bank, the moonlight was with us. A couple of orbits at a safe height of 2,000 feet helped us pick up and discern some of the obstructions around. Doppler and GPS were used for wind and ground speed assessment. A final approach was attempted in a southerly direction. One landing light was focused ahead and the other below to catch any obstructions. All eyes on board had never worked this hard before. The helicopter was brought to hover at 40 metres with reference to the vehicle lights ahead. The wireless tower could be discerned by the furiously flashing torches. A vertical controlled descent brought us down to the ground. After switching off, we could hear the gunfire in the distance.

While the casualties were being loaded, one look at them told us that we had done the right thing. Meanwhile, the crew had a good look around to plan the take-off, which anyway was a less arduous task than the landing. It was only then that we noticed a second defunct wireless tower. The soldiers hadn't bothered about it since the orders or 'hukam' did not mention it. Had we aborted or gone around in our approach, it would have been bang in our path! The take-off was uneventful and the surgeons were waiting when we landed around 10.30 p.m. The doctors worked throughout the night and, to our great satisfaction, all four lives were saved by the morning. More importantly, the BSF officer who had lost one eye while the other was severely damaged by a bullet not only survived but regained partial vision after multiple operations at Sankara Nethralaya at Chennai.

After twenty years, I got a call on my mobile from one Sandeep Mishra. He was the same BSF officer I had saved. He is now completely blind but happily married with a loving family. The BSF had permanently absorbed him as a teaching faculty at their academy in Tekanpur near Gwalior. I had goose pimples as he wept and thanked me after two decades.

### Pasighat in Peril

June was a maddening monsoon month in the year 2000. It was raining the entire month and, on 12 June, tragedy struck Siang district of Arunachal Pradesh in the form of flash floods. Due to a breach and subsequent bursting of an artificial dam caused by a mountain slide in China, water levels in the Siang rose by ten to fifteen metres. A few unlucky souls never got a chance to escape; but to save the rest, the IAF was rushed in. My squadron flew from sunrise to sunset for the next four days and carried out operations from Pasighat, Yingkiong and Along to airlift 2,389 persons, including winching up 265 critical life-and-death cases. The tally of displaced persons included almost 800 schoolchildren stranded away from their homes. For some strange reason, all schools were on the western side of the Siang, while many villages were on the east bank—connected by all kinds of bridges, including ones made of ropes. All these were washed away in the deluge.

The most memorable rescue was made by my gunner, SK. While flying around to locate survivors, something caught his eye. He advised me to go lower to a spot where a figure was just about discernible—the person was all covered in mud and, as we found out on hovering closer, it was a woman submerged in thick mud up to her waist, holding a child up in her arms. We inched closer to her. The only reason she was not blown away was the mud anchoring her. Somehow SK stepped out on the ladder and grabbed the child. The woman was too weak and had given up, but SK hadn't. He removed the stepladder and lay down on the floor with half his body sticking out of the door. Everyone else in the cargo cabin held his legs. Our flight engineer got up to guide me on the radio to get closer. SK held the woman in a strong embrace, while I was guided to slowly go up—literally prising her out of the mud. SK got a presidential gallantry award for such great acts.

We did around 162 challenging missions to deliver 36,720 kg of emergency ration and medicines. At midnight on 12 June, an urgent SOS came from Chief Minister Mukut Mithi, of a steamer having capsized in the swirling waters of the Brahmaputra. In a dramatic rescue from the middle of the river, ninety-eight passengers presumed dead earlier were rescued safely by us from the sinking boat. The other helicopter was captained by Amitabh. Survivors were flown to Pasighat, but on reaching there we found the ALG flooded. I took a split-second decision to divert to Mohanbari, where they were cared for by our base. In recognition of this effort, three unit personnel received gallantry awards. In addition to this, we were also felicitated by the Government of Arunachal Pradesh with Governor's Gold Medal. Incidentally, Amitabh was the captain of the Mi-17 that dropped NSG commandos over Mumbai's Nariman House during the 26/11 attacks. That moment's picture became the face of the courageous act of all those involved in the event.

## Medak Manjra

On 14 September 2008, at 2.30 p.m., as the CO of Helicopter Training School (HTS), I received a message from my HQ that ten people were marooned due to flash floods caused by the release of water from the Singur reservoir, and only an immediate rescue could save their lives. The approximate location of the site was about 40 km west of Medak town—a good half an hour away by helicopter. I got airborne at 3.15 p.m. from Hakimpet, just forty-five minutes after the first warning (on a Sunday), along with Dongre and a newly commissioned officer, Kulkarni, as winch operator.

We proceeded to carry out a search along the Manjra river and towards Nizam Sagar dam. After a brief search, a small temple was located, surrounded by raging flood waters on the other side of the river, opposite the famous Bhavani Temple. There were ten people stranded on a rooftop (terrace), awaiting rescue, and hundreds of people had gathered on the other river bank. During the low recce, a tall tree and numerous wires on poles were observed surrounding the site. The clear area was barely 15x15 feet, making landing impossible. I brought us to a high hover of 20 feet and Kulkarni lowered the rescue cable.

Since the survivors involved were untrained and panicky, they were not able to secure themselves to the rescue strap and damaged it in the process. The rescue strap was then retrieved and the aircraft descended to a height of 10 feet over the terrace with just the bare minimum clearance. This was done in view of the rising river and the limited time available to rescue them before the flood waters took a toll. Thereafter, one by one all survivors were winched up into the aircraft and hauled in by the co-pilot and the winch operator. It was unconventional because they were simply hanging on to the steel cable! After every two survivors were picked up, I proceeded to a paddy field across the river and dropped them off. In all, ten people were lifted to safety in five shuttles. We had flown almost two hours non-stop without landing.

Within a few hours, the then chief minister of Andhra Pradesh, the late Y.S.R. Reddy, rang up to compliment us. The commissioner for disaster relief especially thanked the IAF for the almost-immediate and timely response. In his letter to me, he commended the IAF for this act of courage and professionalism, which the people of Andhra Pradesh would always remember.

## Needle in the Haystack

The chief minister of Andhra Pradesh in 2009 was Y.S.R. Reddy, an extremely powerful and popular politician—also a bulwark of the Congress Party in southern India. The air force base at Hakimpet was notified of the CM's missing helicopter at 1 p.m. on 2 September. The state government provided coordinates that covered a large area, indicating the last possible position. Immediately, two Chetak helicopters from Hakimpet and two helicopters from Bangalore (now Bengaluru) were launched. I was dispatched by Air HQ to the chief secretary's office to be part of the Crisis Management Committee. The state government also requisitioned an Indian Space Research Organization (ISRO) aircraft for photographic runs. The largest search and rescue ever in India, spearheaded by the IAF, was on. Since helicopters could not carry out a search at night due to the weather and the presence of hills, I ensured that a night search continued with SU-30 fighters with infrared pods, which had to undertake air-to-air refuelling to stay up the whole night. Political pressure was immense, with an added presence of four cabinet heavyweights from Delhi—Prithviraj Chauhan, Veerappa Moily, Janardhan Reddy and one more, whose name I cannot recollect. Outside the Secretariat building, thousands maintained a constant vigil and kept up prayers.

By midnight, I realized that the inputs from various sources were confusing and that the area was too large. Incidentally, the last helicopter crash on the Andhra–Jharkhand border took more than forty days to locate, despite a mammoth air and ground search.

Even then, it was a tribal who found the site by chance. I systematically spoke to Air Traffic Control at Chennai and Hyderabad to get authentic radar and last communication inputs. Since the police had access to mobile phones that traversed through various areas covered by the relay towers of various service providers, with the help of a young Greyhound (police commando), I prepared an elaborate overlay of the last-recorded inputs. By sheer innovation and creative thinking, the crisis team was able to prepare a grid of where all the inputs pointed. The time of 9.26 a.m. on 2 September was identified as the point when the helicopter started going down. This was translated into how far it travelled from the last radar position received. A stray SMS received from one of the mobiles in the helicopter at 12.06 p.m., when it was positively on the ground, confirmed the approximate circle of 4-km diameter that we had plotted. I immediately telephoned my pilots at Kurnool at 12.30 a.m. in the night to concentrate only on this circle in the first two hours after sunrise.

The state machinery had more than eight helicopters, offered by various private agencies, to be launched. There was considerable pressure on me to expand the search in terms of the number of helicopters and the area. However, I convinced the four Union ministers and the crisis management team to have faith in the IAF's ability for at least the first two hours on 3 September. The helicopters took off in adverse weather at 6.30 a.m. and headed for the circle. At exactly 8.20 a.m., the wreckage was spotted within the circle. Essentially, any mobile relay station transmits in a cone of 60 degrees. The centre line range goes up to 50 km while the sides cover only about 10 km. What the tower records is the time when any mobile goes off coverage. By sheer ingenuity, this simple information was translated into a most probable position. The police also use this information to track mobile phones of suspects. But this was the first time that a quick pinpointing of a downed aircraft was done.

A huge search operation by more than 5,000 policemen, tens of aircraft and other costly means over an area of hundreds of square kilometres was avoided by the resourcefulness and creative thinking of those in the Secretariat at Hyderabad. It is a moot point that while high-end technology like the ISRO aircraft and SU-30 failed, an idea of correlating mobile inputs succeeded. It goes to show the value of flexible thinking and quick adaptability.

## Messiahs at Mehboobnagar

The first indication of impending trouble in Kurnool district came on 3 September. An SOS was received from the Andhra Pradesh Secretariat, requesting the IAF at Hakimpet to save five schoolchildren from drowning in Mehboobnagar district. About 140 km away from us, in a hamlet called Ashampet, the children were trapped in waist-deep water in the middle of what was two hours earlier a high ground in a small rivulet. They used to cross this daily on their way to school. Suddenly, it was ten times more voluminous. We immediately got airborne, expecting the worst. We reached just half an hour before sunset, to find them in more than waist-deep torrential waters, holding on to each other for their lives. In fact, one small guy had just his head above the water. Not wasting any time, and throwing all rules and procedures to the wind, we started the winching from about 15 feet, since any closer would have blown all of them away. The first one to be picked up was the small guy, while the last boy was the most difficult, since he found it hard to balance himself. There was a huge grateful public and media presence on the other bank—we were on the front pages of newspapers across the country the next day. We, however, did not stop in the dropping visibility but flew back to Hakimpet to land by night.

## Hovering Angels of Kurnool

Unprecedented rains in north Karnataka from 29 September 2009 flooded several districts and cut off areas like Bijapur, Bagalkot and Bellary, with some places receiving over 50 cm of rain in a single day. The floods inundated the Krishna and Tungabhadra rivers. Karnataka released 25 lakh cusecs of water from Almatti and Narayanpur dams in a single day, a record of sorts. With Andhra Pradesh itself in the grip of severe rains in the last week of September, all reservoirs were brimming to their capacities. On 1 October, reports indicated water levels rising dangerously in the town of Mantralayam. They were so high that they submerged most inhabited villages near the riverbank. To say that the situation was critical is an understatement. A village that was about a kilometre away from the riverbank was completely under water. The nearest bank was too far away now and the water level was up to the rooftops. With rising water levels and most people taking refuge on these rooftops, the villagers were not sure whether they were going to survive the next hour or not. Eight helicopters were put under my command to provide relief and rescue operations. My unit's four Chetaks spearheaded the effort.

On 2 October, all four of us got airborne. The task was challenging as operating conditions were critical with the villagers in a dire state—marginal weather made it even worse. On landing at Kurnool, we realized that there was no fuel. The district magistrate approached us with an urgent rescue. A family of thirteen was hanging on for dear life on a rooftop in what now seemed to be the middle of the river—which itself had become a torrential sea with waves. But no helicopter had enough fuel to undertake this mission. I asked for some brand-new, large plastic jerry cans, which materialized in no time. Then, fuel was drained out from the other three choppers to fuel mine. This was not in any book and not permitted, but then these were not normal times. In the meantime, relayed through mobiles, we got news that five members of that family had been washed away, with only a wall left, which the survivors were clinging on to. We reached the spot, and by the time we circled to make the first approach, another three were gone. It was a Herculean task to hover over the raging waters and winch up the remaining five in three shuttles to the nearby bank. There were thousands of villagers gathered on the northern bank since morning, but they had been unable to help out.

The next morning, we all had barely enough fuel for twenty minutes each. To add to the tough conditions, fuel tankers were unable to reach Kurnool due to breaks in the road bridges over the Krishna and the Tungabhadra. So, on one hand, fuel tankers were stuck 20 miles short of Kurnool town and on the other, fuel was mandatory to continue any type of rescue and relief operations. Analysing the gravity of the situation, I got airborne for an assessment sortie (more like a do-or-ditch). A landing spot on the national highway was selected and a decision to operate from NH-7 was taken. The rescue and relief missions continued with the national highway as an airbase for the next two days. Tankers from Hyderabad could reach us there.

In the next few days, in eight rescue missions, we managed to save forty-seven lives that would have surely perished. Each mission was a daunting and challenging experience in itself. The missions varied from picking up people from rooftops to those surviving on trees. In one case, a family of four, comprising husband, wife and two children aged four and six, were stuck on a tree in the centre of the fast-flowing river. It was not an easy task to rescue them from the middle of the tree with all its branches. No orders or procedure existed that specified the manner in which such a mission could be undertaken. We used our ingenuity and experience to hover close by, float the rescue strap on the fast-flowing water towards the tree (à la a kite) and rescue the entire family one by one. This flexible approach took considerable time since it was the survivors who had to understand what we wanted them to do. After their rescue, we noticed that their condition was critical; their skin was totally parched and coming off in flakes. They had been stuck on that tree for over seventy-two hours without food, water and sleep. Every such mission makes helicopter pilots the world over feel proud of their machines.

Half of Kurnool was in two-storey-high floods. People were stuck on rooftops in thousands, and the state government wanted everyone to be rescued! Even if all the helicopters of the IAF had attempted it, this could not have been done. An alternate plan of dropping essential supplies over each roof was made and executed. Almost 1,20,000 kg of relief material, including water, food and medicines were dropped—rooftop by rooftop. This relief was not only a must for their physiological needs, but also, more importantly, to generate a will to survive and provide a ray of hope. Waters started receding by 5 October and boats sent by the state machinery started doing the needful. The entire mission can rightly be summed up in the words of the district collector of Kurnool at a press conference on 7 October, where he stated, 'People of Kurnool will always be indebted forever to the efforts of helicopters of the IAF. Not only did the IAF save forty-seven lives, but it helped thousands every day to believe that survival and help was just around the corner.'

## Heli-Hiccups

A helicopter's ubiquity, or the ability to land virtually anywhere, is a great strength; however, it has its own share of problems, some that can be foreseen and some that are like a bolt from the blue. I remember a train accident in 1985 involving the famous Tinsukia Express. It had happened in the night and I was off with my CO, Bertie, at first light the next day. The place was about 70 km from the refinery at Bongaigaon in Assam. We could easily spot it, not only because of the mess created by the two colliding trains but also by the thousands of onlookers present all around. While rescue efforts were on, so was some looting by unscrupulous persons. We picked up a police party from Bongaigaon, landed in a field next to the crash and switched off.

I stayed near the helicopter while Bertie went to speak to some officials. It seemed that all casualties had been moved by road and there was no immediate requirement from us. We were requested to be available at Bongaigaon. By this time, the police party had disappeared and the crowd, who were mostly refugees from Bangladesh, had started crowding around the chopper. Matters came to a head when they started to touch and possibly try to take away a souvenir! Bertie took a bold decision. He asked me to get in and start the rotors while a seatbelt with a heavy metal quick release box was prised away from the rear seat. This he swirled around shouting at the top of his voice. I saw him landing a few juicy blows while I came to full throttle. He then jumped in and yelled for me to take off—which I did even before he could strap in. It was a close call.

Something similar, but worse, happened when I was a CO in Hakimpet. A cadet and his instructor had just ejected from a Kiran trainer aircraft close to a town named Siddapur. A helicopter with an instructor and his female cadet were diverted from their training to fly to the area. Within ten minutes, I got airborne with a full tank and a doctor on board. The air officer commanding (AOC), a fighter pilot, was in the control tower, giving out instructions on flight radio. The pilots could not be traced near the crash. Actually, they had been picked up by a recently started road ambulance service and taken to a hospital. The AOC asked the first Chetak to land at a college ground in Siddapur. I came on the radio to object, citing crowd issues near a town, but was overruled. Unfortunately, not only did the chopper land but it also switched off to conserve fuel.

By the time we reached them, panic calls had started coming in of people being all over the chopper and the pilots. The lady pilot was repeatedly felt around by some male miscreants. There was only one thing to do. I started doing mock dives at the crowd. I had to come in really low and virtually threaten the crowd with my menacing egg-beater on top—the chopper's rotors. In the meantime, the other chopper started and finally managed to make a run for it. The pilots whom we had come to save returned were finally picked up by an ambulance in the night.

## Countering Insurgency without Choppers? No Way!

The IAF's helicopter fleet has a rich legacy of commitment over decades to fight conflict that is variedly termed as irregular war, counter-insurgency operations or COIN, hybrid wars, sub-conventional operations, less-than-war, and the list goes on. Military history is replete with examples of the weak defeating the strong: Spartans against Athenians; Spanish guerrillas versus the army of Napoleon; Vietnamese Communists against France, and then the United States; and Afghan Mujahideen against the Soviet Union, and then the Americans. The relationship between opponents is asymmetric. In the case of colonial powers, the asymmetric contest is underlined by a total war for the insurgent and a limited one for the 'strong'.

### Darkest Hours

During the dark days of Operation Gibraltar by Pakistan in August 1965, a helicopter task force, initially consisting of two squadrons but later increased to three, was formed to assist in fighting against Pakistani armed infiltrators, or Razakars, who had entered Jammu and Kashmir. This detachment was instrumental in helping the

Indian Army check the influx of more than 15,000 Pakistani raiders and infiltrators. It was mainly based in Srinagar, and it carried out seventy-nine offensive sorties from 20 August 1965 until the end of hostilities. IAF's Mi-4 helicopters, suitably modified, bombed and strafed positions of Razakars in many areas, especially Haji Pir Pass, Tangdhar, Badgam, Mandi, Budil and the hills around Gurez. This was the first time that Indian medium-lift utility helicopters were used in an offensive role, and some unique modifications were done in a matter of days. While these offensive sorties did inflict damage; more importantly, they exerted a great demoralizing effect on Pakistani guerrillas.

## Perennial Problem: The Northeast

Besides the Mizo movement in the Northeast, almost every state among the seven sisters has witnessed different degrees of insurgencies. Nagaland led the way immediately after Independence. Since then, the IAF and Indian air power have played a critical role in supporting governance and conflict management. This synergy with the army and police forces has resulted in innumerable successful operations and fire-fighting scenarios in Nagaland, Tripura, Meghalaya, Assam, Arunachal Pradesh, Mizoram and even peaceful Sikkim, where relief aid had to be flown in when the Gorkhaland agitation in neighbouring West Bengal cut off road connectivity. There are some vivid examples. Hundreds of special heli-borne missions have countered the advantage that terrain affords to the insurgents, besides providing the deterrence threat of a rapid reaction. Some dire contingencies, such as drying up of fuel in Manipur in 2010, were addressed by flying in diesel and petrol in-flight refuelling IL-76s. The development of road and rail networks has been enabled by heavy-lifting of men, material and specialized equipment through a mix of transport aircraft and medium-lift helicopters.

Specialized equipment such as heavy earth movers and trucks has been innovatively heli-lifted to the most far-flung and inaccessible areas by 'breaking' them into manageable packets. Above all, saving the lives of civilians and combatants across the region has been the mainstay of hearts, minds and morale-boosting campaigns.

Logistic support to civilian governance and deployed forces has been the foundation of counter-insurgency in the Northeast for decades. A network of more than a thousand helipads and ALGs across the region enables sustainment as well as rapid reaction to emergent contingencies. Many of these ALGs and forward helipads are manned continuously by IAF detachments, which, over the years, have transformed from rudimentary to modern infrastructure. Virtually every known method of supply by the medium of air has been used to support combat and non-combat efforts to integrate the Northeast into the mainland. Fixed-wing aircraft have carried out air-landed and parachute drops over many decades with venerable aircraft such as Caribous, Otters, Dakotas, Packets and An-32s. Chetak/Cheetahs, Mi-4s, Mi-8s, Mi-17s and the latest V5s have done millions of hours and sorties of para-drop and free drops, and heli-landing in some of the most hazardous, dangerous and difficult terrains of the world. Even the Mi-26, the largest helicopter in the world, has been effectively used for a variety of roles, such as assisting building of infrastructure and supplying critical items at crucial junctures. The hub-and-spoke model of centralized command and decentralized execution of air power has been practised on a daily basis in the Northeast for the last six decades.

The Mizo problem that had been simmering awhile came to a head on the last day of February 1966 when the Mizo National Front (MNF) captured the Aizawl treasury and surrounded the headquarters of 1 Assam Rifles. Other elements of the MNF also surrounded Assam Rifles posts at Champai, Darangaon, Vaphai,

Lungleh and Demagiri across Mizoram. A detachment of six Mi-4 helicopters based at Tezpur was sent to Kumbhirgram airfield on 2 March. On 4 March, attempts were made to fly in soldiers of Assam Rifles, which had been moved to Kumbhirgram from Dimapur, into the besieged post of 1 Assam Rifles in Aizawl. However, the MNF had occupied vantage points north and south of the post and opened fire at the helicopters ferrying in troops. The post fired a red cartridge to indicate that it was not safe for helicopters to attempt a landing. All seven helicopters then returned to Kumbhirgram to await further instructions. One had, in fact, suffered minor damage after taking a bullet on the tail boom.

It is not widely known that Flight Marshal S.H.F.J. Manekshaw, then a lieutenant general and the GOC-in-C Eastern Command, and Air Vice Marshal Y.V. Malse, then the AOC-in-C Eastern Air Command, flew in an IAF Caribou aircraft for reconnaissance over Aizawl. The Caribou limped back to Kumbhirgram airfield riddled with bullet holes. One bullet narrowly missed Manekshaw who, it is understood, was standing behind the co-pilot during the reconnaissance. After consultation with the army and air headquarters, it was decided to fly troops into the 1 Assam Rifles camp with fighter escorts. Accordingly, seven helicopters and four French-built Toofani fighters were used for this operation. The rendezvous was in the Tuirial Valley east of Aizawl. As each helicopter turned on to the final approach towards the makeshift helipad in the Assam Rifles post, one Toofani on each side of the chopper fired rockets at the MNF elements sitting north and south of the post. Suffering casualties, the MNF cadres fled the scene and the siege thus ended. Additional army battalions reached Aizawl by road from Silchar. While Toofanis operating from Kumbhirgram and Hunters operating from Jorhat were subsequently used over Champai, Darangaon, Vaphai and Demagiri, these operations were not coordinated with any helicopter activity. They were undertaken to keep the MNF at bay and to ease the pressure off the surrounded posts till they could be reinforced with troops flown in on a helicopter.

IAF helicopters undertook many quick-reaction operations, including an abortive attempt to raid an MNF camp in erstwhile East Pakistan near the Mizoram border. Mi-4s offered high mobility to troops and a tremendous element of surprise. It was here that the term Special Heli-Borne Operations (SHBO) entered the lexicon of joint army-air force operations of the Indian armed forces. An enemy that had been sitting unchallenged for days or weeks could suddenly, without warning, find itself under assault from troops brought in by helicopters. Pilots had just read about the exploits of similar air mobility operations then ongoing in Vietnam and were willing to undertake such missions, fully confident in their ability. Gen. Sagat's experience with 110 HU perhaps contributed to his confidence in planning for the heli-lifts during the Bangladesh War in 1971, when he headed 4 Corps.

Central Armed Police Forces (CAPFs) are now extensively deployed in situations of widespread terrorism and have acquired considerable experience in counter-insurgency warfare. Although these forces have traditionally worked under the overall command of the army while handling insurgencies in India's Northeast, they have shown remarkable levels of success even when they have been on their own, e.g., operations against Left-Wing Extremists (LWE) in the Red Corridor.

## IAF in Anti-Maoist Operations

It has now been nearly a decade since the IAF was called upon to render support in tackling what has been called the gravest internal threat to India's security. While the initial contribution of the air force as part of Operation Triveni was two helicopters; this was enhanced to four after the Dantewada massacre of April 2010. By the end of 2010, two more helicopters were added to the operation, bringing the total to six. This extended commitment was made possible consequent to the IAF recalling its helicopters from various United Nations missions abroad and the induction of the latest Mi-17 V5 fleet. Currently, Operation Triveni stands as the largest helicopter operation in terms of the area covered with two helicopter squadrons dedicated to provide 24x7 response and support to the CAPFs, state police forces and the administration.

On 14 November 2008, an IAF helicopter was tasked to carry out election duties at Jagdalpur in Chhattisgarh. It flew fifty-eight sorties, airlifting 215 passengers and 2,905 kg of load in Naxalite-affected areas. In keeping the democratic process of elections alive, the unit lost one air warrior when the helicopter came under fire from the Naxalites during take-off. The crew showed exemplary courage and presence of mind in taking evasive action and, despite the loss of one crew member and a damaged aircraft, flew back to safety, saving the lives of twelve passengers. This act also denied a source of propaganda to the anti-national elements. A four-helicopter detachment at Jharkhand for election duties in November and December 2009 was instrumental in its success. As many as 475 sorties were utilized for airlifting 16 tonnes of load and 3,741 passengers. Apart from the main role of airlifting polling parties, the IAF also carried out numerous casualty evacuations and area-domination sorties in affected areas.

## Operation Triveni

As the threat from Naxalites continued to grow and turned out to be the single largest internal threat to the country by the end of 2009, the IAF was tasked with supporting counter-insurgency operations in coordination with paramilitary forces and civil police in the Red Corridor. Four helicopters were deployed at Raipur and Jagdalpur from December 2009 to September 2011. Operations were undertaken in a large geographical area comprising eight states, making it one of the largest sustained helicopter operations ever undertaken by the IAF. All helicopters were configured with door- and blister-mounted guns manned by IAF commandos or Garuds. The IAF also undertook training of paramilitary forces so as to carry out seamless coordinated missions.

From the outset, the Indian government has been unequivocal in its stand that IAF assets will only be employed in a support role with no direct offensive application in any form. Consequently, in spite of the tremendous firepower at hand, the IAF has employed its helicopters only in reinforcing troops, evacuating casualties, providing air logistics support to those deployed on ground, besides carrying out aerial reconnaissance over hilly and mountainous areas of this region. The operation mainly covers the states of Chhattisgarh, Bihar, Jharkhand, Maharashtra, Andhra Pradesh and Orissa.

Earlier constrained by a series of mine and improvised explosive device (IED) blasts, CAPFs have now been able to increase their footprint over a larger area, as their reliance on roads as the sole means of supplies has gradually reduced. Over the more than 15,250 hours and 20,000 sorties flown by the IAF in Operation Triveni, it has been able to airlift 1,600 tonnes of load and 90,000 troop rotations. Needless to say, ferrying this load over mine-ridden roads would have entailed a great degree of danger and vulnerability. The ability to fly in reinforcements during ongoing operations has also allowed a high tempo of operations over a longer period of time than was possible. An example is the operation conducted in Gaya in September 2016, where CAPFs were able to maintain their pursuit of LWE in a remote region, primarily due to the fact that men and material could be flown in with alacrity. Since then, many such 'carrying the battle to the opponent' missions have been done, breaking the back of the extremist movement.

Such operations are now conducted with the knowledge that casualties, if any, would be extracted promptly by IAF helicopters. The effect of this knowledge on a soldier's morale has a telling effect on his performance during operations. The IAF has evacuated more than 1,200 casualties so far. Retrieval of almost 500 mortal remains by day and night has shown the commitment to bring each soldier back. Once again, during the operation in the Gaya region, eight casualties were recovered by the IAF in spite of inclement weather, bullets flying all around and no regular helipad in the vicinity of the operation. By going into this area repeatedly during the operation, aircrew displayed their commitment to the cause at hand.

There are numerous such instances wherein the IAF contributed gainfully to operations on the ground. In June 2008, an IAF helicopter crew on a flood relief mission in West Bengal was tasked with recovering a party of policemen engaged in a fire fight with insurgents in Malkangiri district. On that fateful day, sixty-two policemen were travelling in a boat near Balimela dam in Malkangiri district to augment the fighting force at a police post. The party was ambushed and came under heavy fire. Out of the team of sixty-two, only eight survived while continuing to be surrounded by heavily armed guerrillas. After detailed planning, these survivors were safely evacuated by IAF helicopters.

The criticality of the IAF in ground operations was also evident when, after the infamous Dantewada incident where more than seventy-five troops were killed by LWEs, two IAF helicopters brought in reinforcements near Chintalnar, which prevented any further attacks. Much later, on 17 December 2010, a massive ground operation was launched by Special Forces of the Andhra Pradesh police—the Greyhounds—which resulted in the killing of four Maoists and the capture of another five. However, the

Greyhounds got stuck for want of rations and ammunition, and for final extraction. Two helicopters were launched from Jagdalpur to extract more than 130 Greyhound troops from the thick jungles of Andhra Pradesh, north of Narayanapatnam. The operation was carried out from makeshift clearings in the jungles. The mission was a huge success in boosting the morale of the Greyhound battalion.

These operations, however, can be hindered by numerous problems, with certain combinations proving to be extremely hazardous. The natural combination of monsoons over hilly and wooded terrain makes helicopter flying in this region very challenging to say the least. Flying for extended periods in such an environment without any radio contact and ground radar contact adds to the hazards faced by IAF aircrew on a daily basis. Added to this mix is the ever-improving arsenal of the extremists. Besides acquiring light machine guns (LMGs) and rocket-propelled grenades (RPGs), extremists are also educating themselves on how to engage with helicopters better. A booklet called 'Guerrilla Air Defence' has been included in the syllabus that an LWE has to study. Consequent to these efforts, extremists have been able to hit four aircraft—in one case with fatal consequences. The IAF has consequently been revising its procedures, laying certain strictures to prevent a recurrence of any mishap. Military history is replete with examples where operations over a long haul tend to cater to the law of averages while one-time affairs are brasher. Operating from non-military airfields and the danger to IAF helicopters on the ground also remains a constant worry for planners.

Irrespective of the dangers involved, aircrew have placed upon themselves very restrictive rules of engagement, which treat the entire operation as being one against an insurgency, rather than against terrorists. This distinction ensures that IAF helicopters fire only in self-defence, and that too not from any of their integral heavy weapons but from sideward-facing LMGs. Proportionality and avoiding collateral damage is thus built into operations. In addition to the mammoth task that the IAF has accomplished towards this operation, officers and soldiers of the IAF have also trained more than 2,000 police personnel in various special ops, including slithering operations, low hover jumps and air maintenance. A large number of ground training programmes have also been conducted for paramilitary forces. The focus is on making these troops proficient in undertaking weather assessment, handling radio communication and being capable of efficient load planning. The detachment has also been undertaking numerous missions of troop insertion and extraction in the Red Corridor region.

To further enlarge the CAPF footprint, pre-positioning of aviation fuel in certain areas has been ensured, thus increasing the radius of action. Most established helipads have been upgraded to accept night-vision goggle-enabled sorties. The employment of helicopters has acted as a force multiplier and given a huge impetus to anti-Naxal operations of the paramilitary forces. The mere presence of helicopters is a source of strength to troops as it provides much needed logistic/communication back-up, recce/observation capability, life-saving missions, timely augmentation of troops and any other special requirements. In short, Operation Triveni has been a huge enabler and morale booster for paramilitary forces. In the period that they have been part of these operations, IAF helicopter pilots have upheld their reputation as being true saviours from the sky. The synergy between the IAF and police forces is at the core of the successful turnaround in operations in the Red Corridor.

# VIDESHI MELEE (MELA!)

THIS SECTION IS a tribute to the people of Africa in general, and the Congolese in particular. Despite facing great historical wrongs at the hands of colonizers, and the adversity of war-like conditions since then, these simple people epitomize the resilience of the human race. As a Blue Helmet or UN Peacekeeper, one sees this stark reality first-hand. Congo (officially the Democratic Republic of the Congo) is the worst, and that's where the Indian choppers did yeoman service post 2003 to support civilian protection.

These stories are about combat against militia who neither understood nor respected any rules and norms about civil liberties and the value of human life. The tales paint the horrors of brutal tactics such as rape as a weapon of war and the use of child soldiers. But they also bring out many positives and the fun side of operating in the Congo. That spells hope for the Congolese.

## Preparing for MONUC

When we were preparing our contingent for the UN Mission in the Congo (MONUC is an acronym based on its French name), the chief of air staff (fondly called Kitcha) one day called in all the three commanders, i.e., Gill, Sunil and me, for a long-drawn-out session. His main theme was that all earlier IAF sojourns with the UN had ended abruptly and never lasted more than a year. He described in detail the adventures of IAF Canberras in the early 1960s, Somalia (1992–93) and Sierra Leone (1999). All IAF detachments had to leave in a hurry before completing their tenure. His refrain was to display commitment and effectiveness of such high standards that the world in general and the UN in particular would sit up and take notice. Kitcha was emphatic that heads would roll if our mission did not fare better than the previous ones.

With that message and a starting line-up that boasted the best in human and material resources of the service, we were all set to go. My other book on peacekeeping missions captures the full details; however, by the time we finished in August 2004, the UN wanted us to stay for longer. Not only did our Goma mission continue for the next eight years, another one in Bukavu, one in Kindu and one in Sudan also sprang up. We defined robustness in peacekeeping like never before. All these detachments were wound up in 2011 by the Indian government because of operational commitments in combating left-wing extremism over vast swathes of our own country. Imagine, I started the MONUC detachment as a commanding officer and finally wound it up as a principal director in Air HQ. What a complete circle!

### Kirtan at Kigali

We were first deployed from New Delhi to Kigali by air, the site of a famous genocide museum dedicated to the victims of the 1994 massacre of mainly Tutsis by the Hutus. A visit there shakes one up. Rows and rows of skulls and other displays drive home the reality of how cruel men can get when aroused by racial or tribal passions. It is an apt and iconic dedication to 'Lest We Forget'.

It took thirteen An-124 (the giant Russian plane) sorties to completely deploy us. The huge plane is managed by a small crew trained to handle standard cargo containers with motor winches, pulleys and cables. Similarly, at Kigali there was only one crane operator and eight drivers of flat-top trucks that were to be loaded with containers. Somewhere and somehow, they forgot to tell us about containers. We had just arrived at Palam, Delhi, in trucks with an assortment of thousands of individually well-packed items varying in size, as much as one could imagine. The An-124 crew just gave up, told us to load however we wanted to and went to rest in their hotel rooms. They came back at midnight to secure the entire load and took off, still shaking their heads.

In Kigali, for the first hour, UN drivers and the crane operator, in complete disbelief, refused to touch anything. Fortunately, our passenger plane carrying half the contingent also landed. All hands on deck and a great deal of sweating ensured loading and securing of the entire load to the flat-tops. That, and the offloading at Goma, made it the toughest day that we went through in our entire stay, which included actual combat! We learnt our lessons, and urgent calls ensured emergency and rapid procurement of containers in Delhi for subsequent flights.

## Saving the Congo

Indian Air Force Contingents (IACs) in UN missions truly stood tall among all others in the business of peace. Many do not publicly acknowledge this for many reasons, but deep inside know that the will and professionalism displayed by the IAF's air warriors was second to none. Even the Indian Army, deployed since decades, has gone through its ups and downs, including scathing criticism at times. But report after report, UN-sponsored or independent, concedes that even before 'robustness' became a fashionable word with the publication and debate surrounding UN doctrines like 'Capstone' and initiatives like 'New Horizon', none ever found the IACs wanting in robustness—it all had to do with ethos, ethics and air warrior-like qualities. India has been one of the staunchest supporters of the United Nations and the multilateralism it represents. No other single idea or organization has contributed more to reducing conflicts in the world in the last six decades. The most visible face of the UN at the grassroots level is its peacebuilding endeavours, a major prerequisite and constituent of which is the entire gamut of peacekeeping.

As the situation in northeast Congo turned grave with repeated massacres of innocent civilians, the international community decided to strengthen military presence there. In July 2003, the second engagement of the IAF after 1961 started in the Congo. In 2003, the IAF was to provide Mi-17 utility helicopters, along with Mi-25 attack helicopters phase-wise, to be based at Goma and Bunia as Indian Aviation Contingent-I. Encouraged by the difference we made, the UN followed it by setting up an Indian Airfield Support Unit at Kindu in Maniema Province in September 2004. With further encouraging results, the Security Council authorized MONUC to add more teeth to its already formidable military air arm by inducting night-capable Mi-17s and night-upgraded Mi-35s as part of Indian Aviation Contingent-II at Bukavu in the South Kivu Province in February 2005. These invaluable assets increased MONUC's credibility to enforce peace in eastern Congo, and it was able to reach areas that had so far been outside its sphere of influence.

My personal inspiration to put my heart and soul into peacekeeping was a chance reading of *King Leopold's Ghost* (1998) by Adam Hochschild, which documents the misrule of the Belgian king that resulted in unmatched cruelty, slavery and deaths (above 10 million) from 1885 to 1908, in just twenty-three years. It makes Leopold one of the greatest tyrants on earth. Almost every officer of my squadron was made to read this, and we all were moved; but the saga continues even as I write. The title of the book is extracted from a poem titled 'The Congo' by Vachel Lindsay, in which Leopold's actions are condemned.

*Listen to the yell of Leopold's ghost*
*Burning in Hell for his hand-maimed host*
*Hear how the demons chuckle and yell*
*Cutting his hands off, down in Hell.*

Casualties suffered are a good measure of the difficulties encountered in an operation. Missions with high casualty levels have been among the least successful. Among UN missions, the Congo has the highest number of casualties, reflecting the nature of the operation. After the Congo, operations in Cambodia, lightly manned as a proportion of the population, had the highest casualty level, followed by Sierra Leone. The experience of the Indian Aviation Contingent over eight years (2003–11) in the Democratic Republic of the Congo brought out one stark lesson that stood above all others: that the legitimacy of peace operations had to be fundamentally based on protecting people. And, in a peacekeeping environment, they had to rely on credible deterrence with severely limited resources on ground.

### Mi-17s: UN Lifelines

Equatorial Eagles, the Mi-17 squadron that I commanded in 2003–04, commenced operations in July 2003. Very we soon realized that flying in this desolate country was not everyone's cup of tea. Though our duties remained essentially what we had been executing back home, the going was never easy with nature playing a big role in making things trickier than they should have been. It threw unique challenges at the aircrew in terms of both weather and terrain; rain, clouds and turbulence are regular companions on most sorties in the Congo. To make matters worse, the area is littered with mountains and volcanoes that stretch across the Great Rift Valley. As any aviator would agree, mountains and bad weather make a very heady mix that is best avoided. Mention must be made here of the hundreds of aircraft of various hues and colour that flew around in an uncontrolled sky, doing all kinds of illegal work—also, the stench of vodka ran high around the pilots of these planes! If the skies were unfriendly, the thick foliage below made the thought of any in-flight emergency rather scary, to say the least. The thick jungle canopy had three different layers of ecosystems within it. But for the Congolese love for the game of soccer and the attendant fields of various sizes and shapes, we would have had very few places to land on. The combined wisdom based on experience in India's Northeast allowed us to devise procedures that ensured operations without any major compromise to flight safety.

This baptism by fire ensured that we got into the groove quickly. Flying tasks ranged from mundane passenger and cargo sorties to missions like troop insertion/extraction under hostile fire, logistic support, communication, medical and casualty evacuation. We moulded into the international environment, displaying exemplary collaboration with other contingents—the common objective being protection of civilians. All peace initiatives and processes adopted by our two brigades were quite ably supported. With changes in the mandates of MONUC involving joint operations with Congolese troops, the squadron revised its standard operating procedures and tactics to mitigate risks with relatively untrained troops. This included removing all live rounds from rifles before embarking. During one such operation, we inducted 146 Congolese troops in sixteen sorties, utilizing all the five helicopters within a short duration of four hours. For our good work in support of ground operations, we were awarded a unit citation by the force commander of MONUC, a first at that point of time.

## Mi-25s: UN Lifeguards

While Mi-17s provided a non-violent element, attack helicopters, nicknamed Vipers, projected the aggressive edge of the Blue Helmets. It was said that the militia in Congo was afraid of only two things in this world—God and an attack helicopter. This was vividly seen in convoy support missions where the mere moving of the front gun turret ensured that militiamen ducked for cover. Vipers with their credo of 'lethal when provoked' were kept busy, mostly in the Ituri sector, providing support to UN ground troops and utility helicopters. There were hundreds of occasions for effective fire support to be provided in dire situations. Post-attack assessment by UN troops almost always revealed considerable damage inflicted to the militia, both to their muscle and morale. During the period of deputation, Vipers carried out missions like escorting Mi-17s carrying ground troops, combating air patrols to ground operations, and showing of force and area domination missions in support of various campaigns.

## Bunia Bedlam

Before our actual deployment in May 2003, I had gone to the Congo as part of an advance party to assess suitability of infrastructure for inducting our contingent. While the main discussions took place in Kinshasa, a trip was planned to the farthest north-east district of Ituri, which happened to be the most disturbed of all. I landed in a small UN aeroplane along with the head of MONUC. As we drove through the streets of Bunia, an almost eerie calm was pervasive.

The dominant militia had lined up child soldiers armed to the teeth all through the 5 km drive. All of them had glazed looks in their eyes, as if looking through you—quite obviously, they had been heavily drugged.

On arrival at the MONUC HQ at Bunia, which was heavily fortified and guarded by soldiers from Uruguay, I got a sense of being completely hemmed in. Uruguayan soldiers, as I found out later, had been recruited from the streets just three months back and looked untrained and unmotivated—ready to run at the first shot. And that is exactly what had been happening for the last few months. Since most UN staffers were Africans and locals, they were extremely vulnerable and did not venture out of the camp. In the meeting with the MONUC head, the hall was full of people with complaints of near-death events. I was introduced with a mention that Indian attack helicopters were coming in. The entire crowd cheered and clapped and, in fact, lapsed into a song-and-dance routine at the hint of 'real' protection. This came from the experience of the ruthless use of attack helicopters by earlier powers that be. We had to leave in a hurry because of intelligence from Kinshasa that chaos was imminent. On landing at Kinshasa, a bullet hole was discovered in our plane. In fact, the situation worsened to such a level in a week that France had to deploy its armed forces till we arrived with our entire might two months later.

Even after we were actually deployed in Bunia in July 2003, with severe restrictions on firing, the mere presence of a Mi-25 sent all belligerents into hiding. However, for a long time there was no actual firing, except for warning shots, because of UN bureaucratic procedures. I thought it was more to do with self-preservation because of the fear of all hell breaking loose. They insisted that every firing had to have clearance and would inevitably be followed by an inquiry. But one day in late 2003, the HQ started getting surrounded by a certain militia group and its leader who put up a challenge in

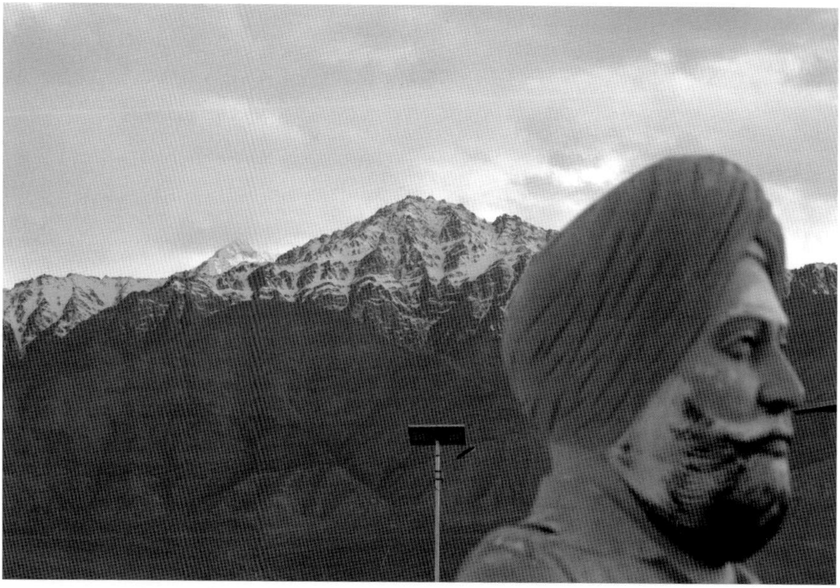

The bust of IAF Air Commodore Mehar Singh, who was nicknamed Baba, at the Leh airbase, and the peak in the background is named after him

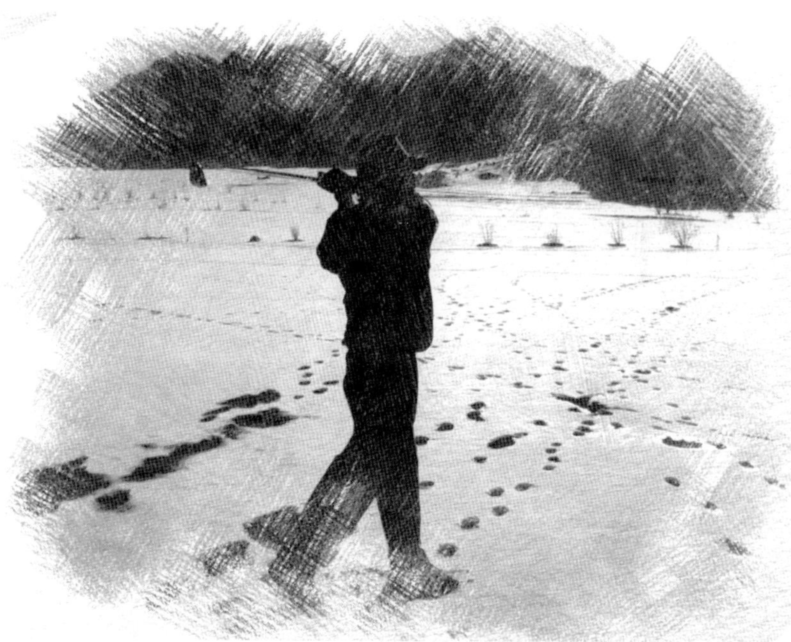

The author playing a round of golf at the Leh army golf course at 13,000 ft and minus 25 degrees Celsius

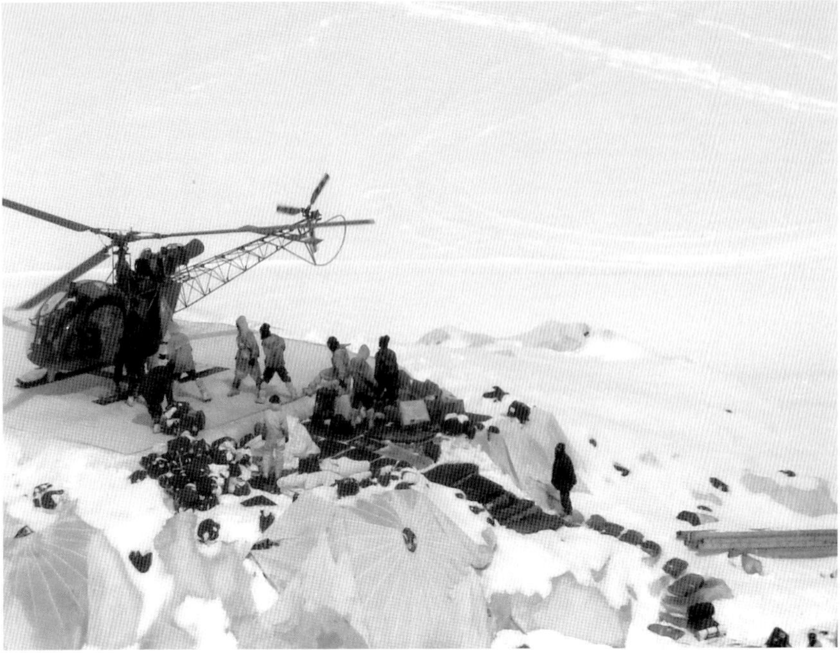

A Cheetah on the Siachen glacier during an aerial resupply and support mission

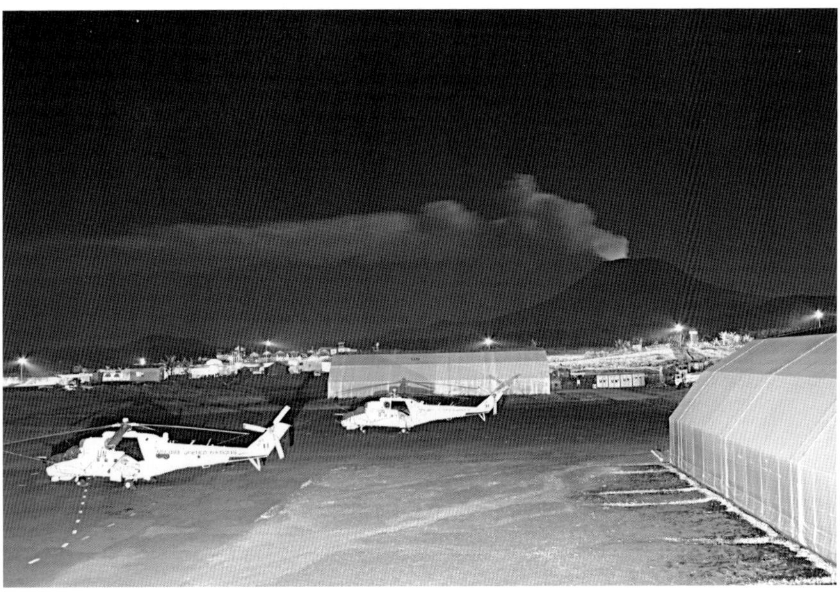

At Goma, North Kivu, in the Congo, a few nights before Mount Nyiragongo erupted in 2004

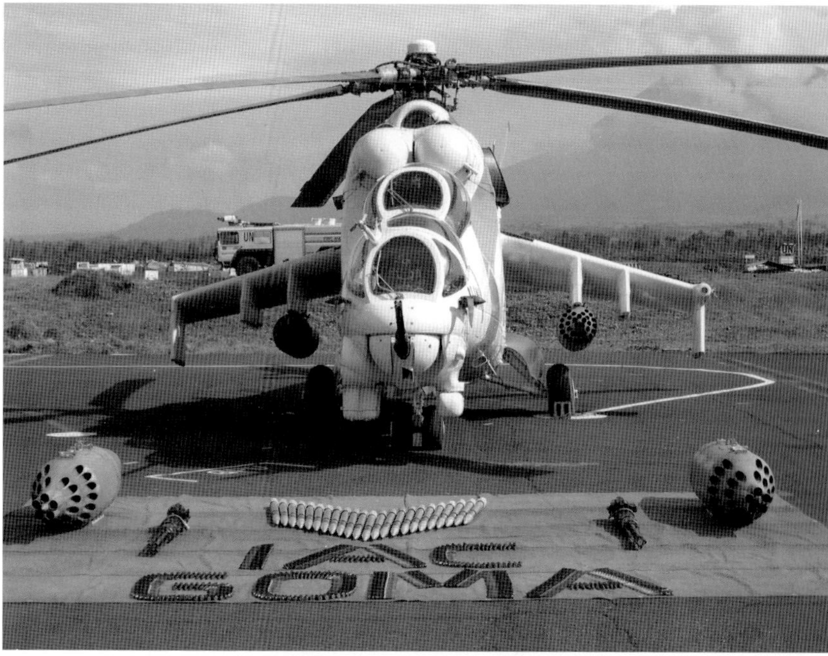

A lethal Mi-25 showing off its prowess in UN white

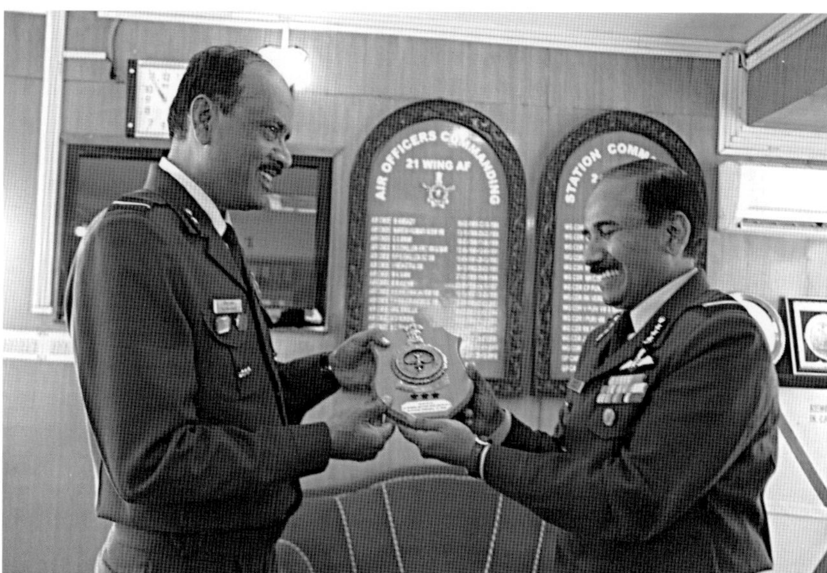

Air Chief Marshal Arup Raha, Chief of the Air Staff, on his first visit to Leh in January 2014

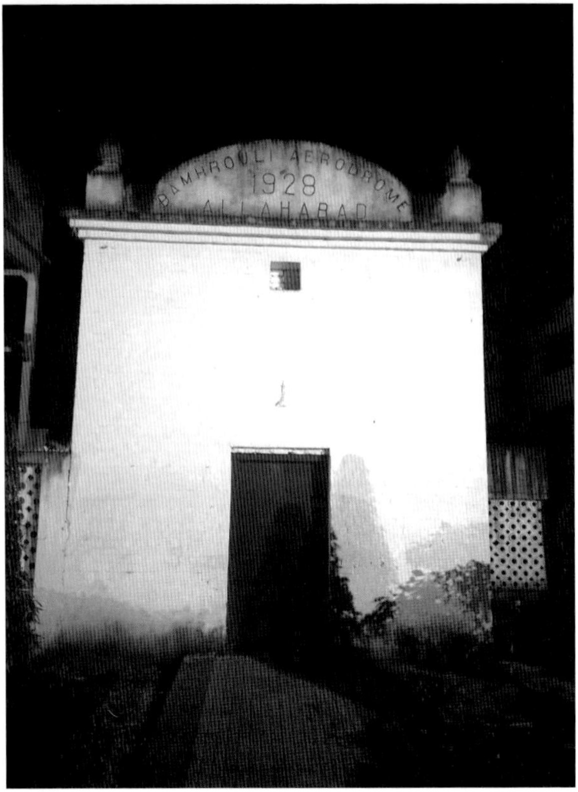


The original air terminal in Allahabad (now Prayagraj), established in 1928

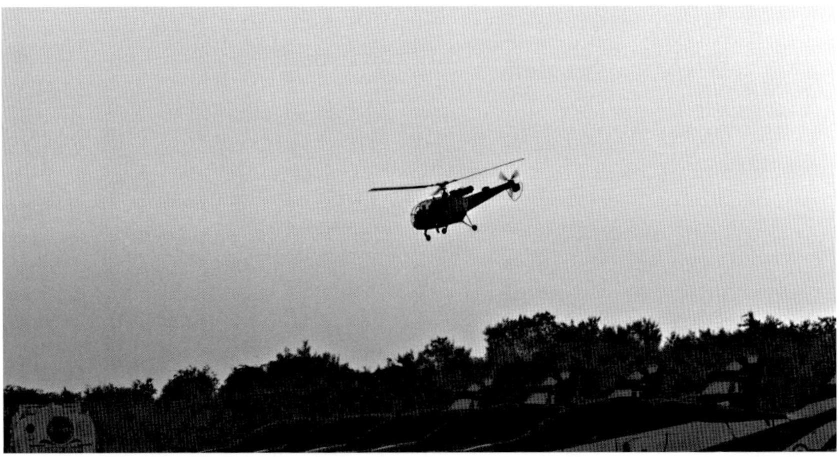

The Alloutte (Chetak), which was a workhorse for the IAF for sixty years

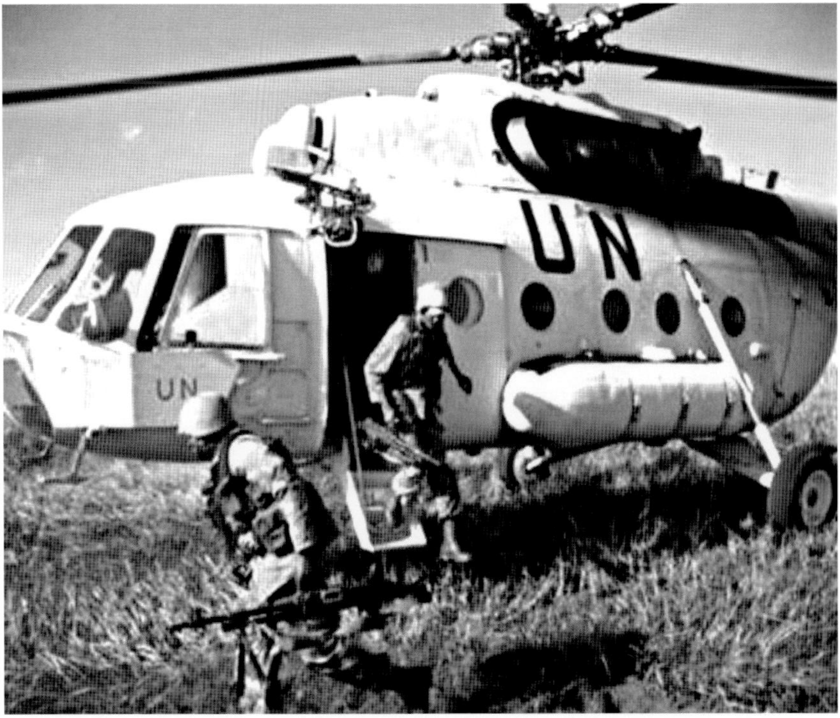

The Blue Helmets (UNPK soldiers) alighting from a Mi-17 during an operation against the Congo militia

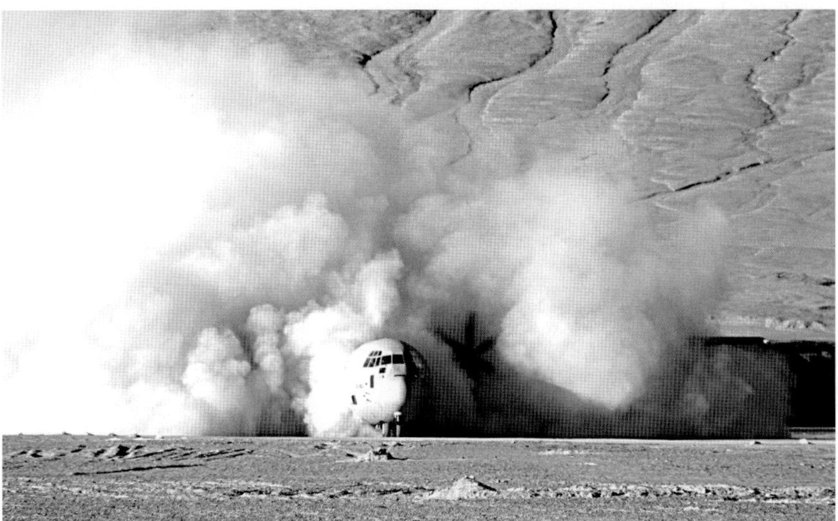
The first landing of a C-130 in Daulat Beg Oldie in Ladakh on 21 August 2013

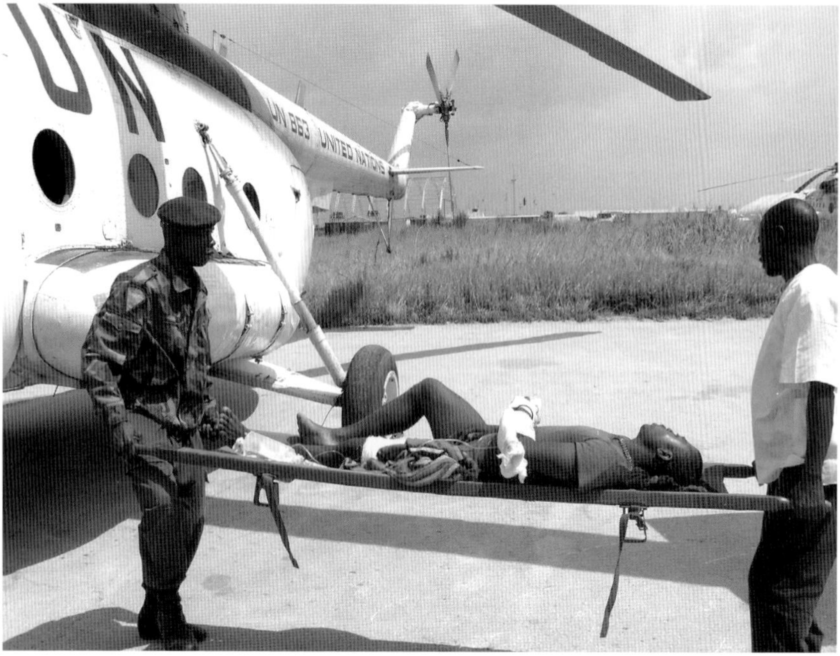


A wounded Congolese army soldier being air-evacuated from the battlefield

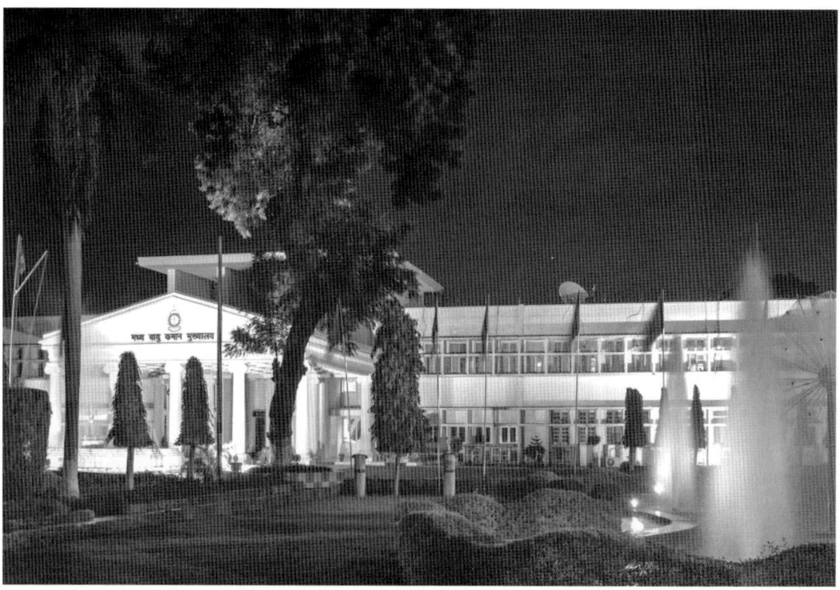

The imposing headquarters of the Central Air Command in Prayagraj

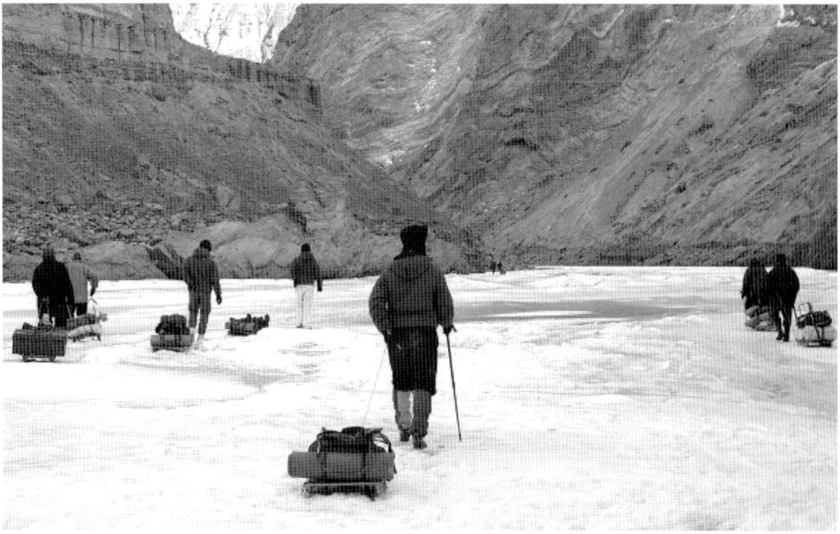

The author (centre) with the IAF team of Leh on the 'Chadar' in the Zanskar valley

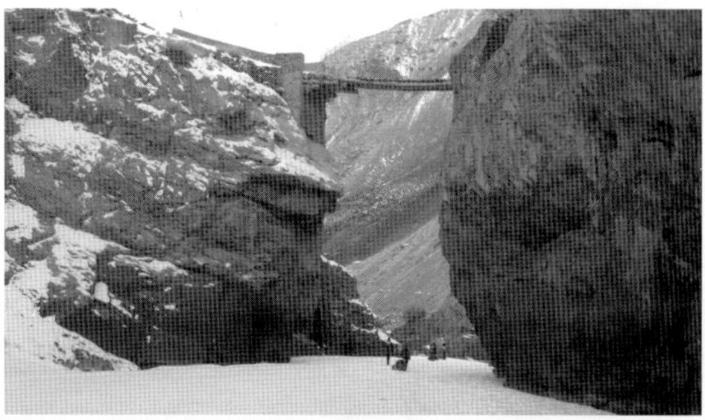

A view of the Chadar trek with Niraq as the backdrop

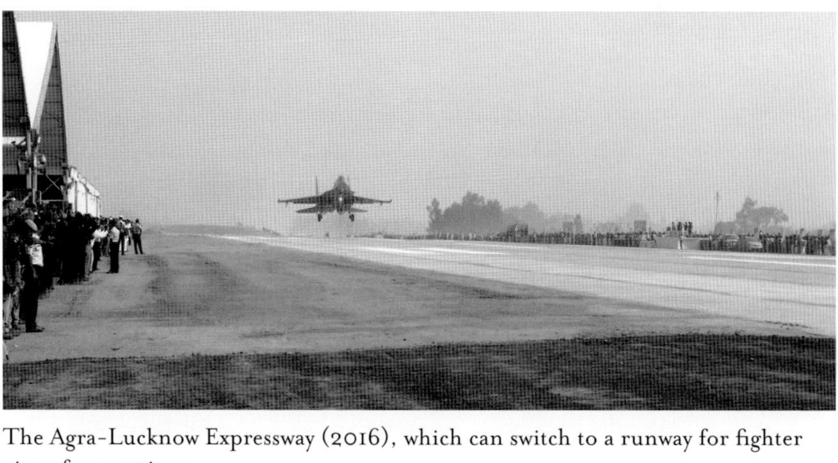

The Agra-Lucknow Expressway (2016), which can switch to a runway for fighter aircraft operations

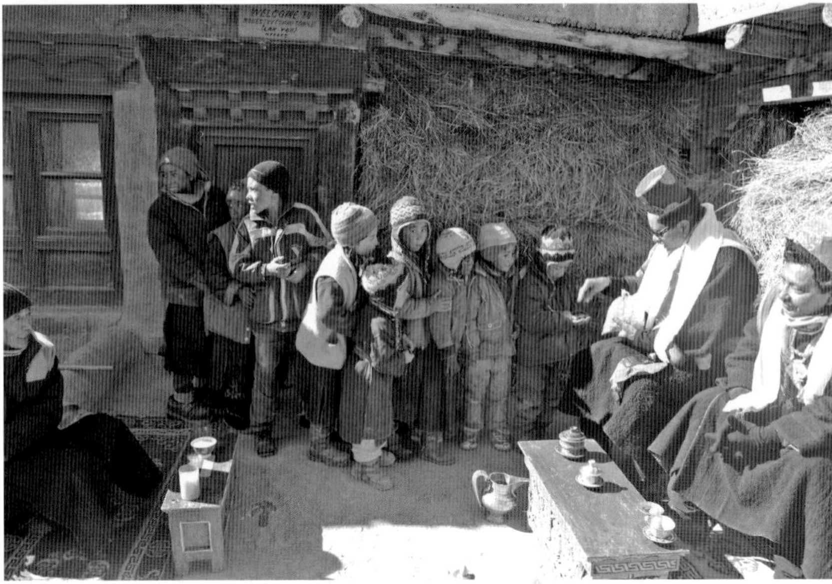

The author distributing sweets to a few children in Niraq

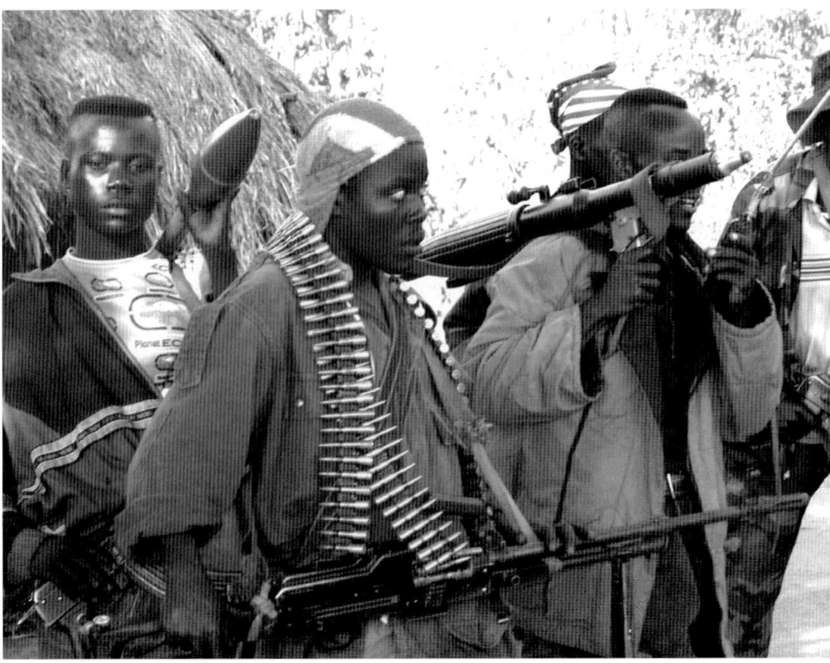

A few Congo rebel militia men armed to the teeth

an extremely menacing way—quite obviously he perceived it as a do-or-die situation. The whole camp was surrounded and the leader was going up and down the road in his open jeep, daring the UN in front of the entire town. A couple of the militiamen fired at the wall of the compound. That did it—a Mi-25, which had buzzed earlier as a warning, aimed at the vehicle and let go a burst of just three rounds. Two of them found their mark, including one that went through the leader's heart! The entire militia army melted away faster than a slab of butter on a hot flame. While the element of chance and good luck was not lost on the pilots, the legendary marksmanship of IAF pilots became the talk of the Congo for years.

### Mount Nyiragongo

This is a majestic volcano overlooking Goma town. Just before we arrived in 2003, it had erupted and taken out half of Goma with its lava, including a large part of the airfield and runway. Our operations used to take place on what was left of the airfield. So inspiring and breathtaking was the view of Nyiragongo from there that we decided to trek up to the top. We had heard that volcanologists had been going up. So, one fine Sunday, fifteen of us attempted the arduous climb. Lush tropical growth gave way to sparser and more unique flora as we approached the top. The view into the crater inspired awe—clouds of sodium and a fiery red ball. Just like a bomb ready to go off. And go it did, in 2004. It began at night and what a sight it was; but Goma was not in danger since the lava flow was northwards. We flew many sorties with volcanologists to study it from a closer range. Sometimes, you could get the pungent smell in the cockpit. During the Bukavu crisis in 2004, a team of volcanologists was kidnapped for ransom from the top. Somehow, they managed to send a message out before that. We planned a rescue mission with a Mi-17, preceded by a Mi-25, which did some menacing dives. The militia fled and I picked up the team with a low hover from the solidified lava near the summit since it was not possible to land. It was a fitting tribute to the beautiful Nyiragongo.

### Shabunda Show of Strength

One of the first operations—and what later became a landmark—took place around Shabunda. A situation was unfolding in this remote town where gold and diamond were mined. Apparently, no MONUC member had set foot in the area for the last two years. That last attempt had resulted in all Milobs (military observers) and helicopter crew being manhandled and kept as hostages for three days. So we were breaking new ground for MONUC. This time around, the UN had the muscle to do it; muscle in the form of a Mi-17 escorted by a Mi-25—the former piloted by me and Marchi, and the latter by Allen and Dutta. Armed with a loaded front gun and two full rocket pods, Allen overtook us 4 km short of the airfield and buzzed through the town of Shabunda. Once he was sure that all appeared to be okay, he gave the all-clear for us to land. As we landed, four South African troops jumped out and took positions on the periphery. Another four got down and took positions around the Mi-25. When all appeared to be calm, save the milling denizens of Shabunda, four Milobs got down and drove off for negotiations. While they were away, a small fixed-wing aircraft showed up on the approach to the runway, which had two helicopters parked on one end of the landing ground. But the aeroplane landed, stopped short, disgorged its load and took off in the other direction—all with the two helicopters still parked on the landing ground! Meanwhile, the local Mayi-Mayi militia leader wasn't willing to play ball and was peeved at not having been informed of the landings. So, the Milobs got in and returned to Kindu. But the intent and resolve of the UN had been shown. A few weeks later, after an even more deadly deployment, the Mayi-Mayi leader relented and agreed to compromise.

## Bukavu Belligerence

The main protagonist in the crisis of Bukavu in 2004 was General Nkunda, who had been accused of having masterminded the assassination of Laurent Kabila, the erstwhile President. He used to reside in Goma, under the protection of General Obedi, commander of the Ninth Military Region (Goma Area), who was also his brother-in-law. Nkunda had consistently refused Kinshasa's offers of a posting in the capital city, citing 'personal security' as the reason. However, it was well known that his role in the assassination and earlier massacres in Kisangani were the real reason for him not wanting to go to Kinshasa. His errant behaviour in the past had led MONUC to believe that he was playing a dirty game. He continued to jockey for a more powerful position to get himself absolved of his past crimes. A Congolese, with part-Tutsi parentage, he was a known Rwanda supporter and was believed to be colluding with the Rwandan army in an effort to foment trouble in the Kivus. Past reports had indicated that the Rwandan army's chief of staff, General James Kabare, had slipped into the Congo on 6 or 7 February 2004 to meet with General Nkunda. The meeting terminated with the two agreeing to accelerate the execution of an agenda. MONUC feared that this meeting could be a harbinger of the third rebellion.

Rwandans had always seen eastern Congo as a part of its own country, denied to them by their former colonial rulers. On 4 May, President Kagame of Rwanda went so far as to issue a statement saying that he wouldn't shy away from sending troops into Congo. In other words, he was prepared to use rebel commanders as a means to achieving his aim of integrating eastern Congo into Rwandan borders. This region has two prominent towns, namely Goma and

Bukavu. While Bukavu is the capital of South Kivu district, the HQ of MONUC's Kivu Brigade Force was at Goma, the capital of North Kivu and the HQ of Rwandan-backed rebel groups. In addition, MONUC's military assets, including our helicopters, were based in these two towns. Control of the axis between the two was thus seen as a major prerequisite to controlling the region. The towns are connected by a solitary road, besides the ferry route across Lake Kivu. Any retreat by Nkunda would be seen as a loss of face, making the current stand-off effectively his last attempt at gaining power (actually, he continued trying right till 2010).

Hostilities broke out on the evening of 26 May in Bukavu, when elements loyal to Nkunda clashed with other units of the Congolese army. Accordingly, following a request by MONUC authorities, we were prepared for an early-morning take-off the next day. A Mi-25 was launched to carry out an aerial recce over the town. It reported heavy small arms and mortar fire from some sections of the town. News reports after the day's fighting cited ten to fifteen people having died in the firing. Another Mi-25 was dispatched to the Bukavu airfield, while one was recalled from Bunia to augment the two in Goma. The former carried out another armed recce/show of force over the town, before returning to Bukavu. These helicopters were in constant touch with UN ground troops in the city, including one of them acting as a forward air controller. In addition, four Mi-17s were also sent to Bukavu airfield, from where they inserted a company of UN troops into a stadium in the town. Since the UN HQ was under fire, helicopters could not land on the helipad that was pinned down by rebels with a well-placed heavy machine gun. The inducted troops later proved to be instrumental in reinforcing the beleaguered UN HQ, where all the local staff had gathered. I carried out an emergency medical evacuation sortie under fire, recovering a female NGO worker with a gunshot wound. All Mi-17 operations were carried out with top cover from the

Mi-25, which subsequently took out the militia machine gun with its front cannon.

## Silverback Serenity

Virunga National Park, established in 1925, is the oldest among Africa's great parks developed to preserve wildlife. But the civil war starting in 1991, and other conflicts continuing until almost 2012, decimated the wildlife in the whole park. The park covers the area around volcanoes such as Nyiragongo, areas next to Rwanda housing the famous mountain gorillas, and large sectors north and south of Lake Edward with exotic pygmies, Tongo chimpanzees and the elusive okapi. Especially after the 1994 Rwanda genocide, almost a million refugees and armed groups were forced to live off the land and animals in these reserves, causing catastrophic environmental degradation. Along with some colleagues, I made a day trip to Virunga, to the abode of the mountain gorilla. The 'gentle giants' were mesmerizing, but so was the commitment and dedication of the park rangers and the many individuals who risked life and limb so that this legacy could be preserved. Over the years, as peace prevailed, hippo and elephant strengths have increased, and there is hope ahead. In the north, beyond Lake Edward, are the distant snow-clad Rwingru Mountains at 16,000 feet. Yes, Congo has snow too, just like Mount Kilimanjaro in Kenya!

## Couldn't-Care-Less Aviation

Technical practices followed by freelance Russians in the Congo were eye-openers. While the UN had hired a few Ukrainian Mi-8s (actually souped-up Mi-17s with extra endurance), the local army also had one Mi-8 along with four fixed-wing aircraft (An-26, two An-28s and An-32). To support these aircraft, there were all of seven ground crews, with only one qualified to work on the chopper! One day, this Russian Superman was faced with a leaking dragging hinge on the main rotor hub—a humungous technical problem. Not one to be cowed down by the enormity of the task, he removed all five blades (without a crane) assisted by just four Congolese workers (not qualified to handle these, obviously). And then he went on to remove the hub—all virtually single-handed. For those watching, it was a lesson in the brilliant use of ropes, levers and pulleys. Of the pilots, the lesser said the better. Their operations had most of us standing by with our hearts in our mouths. Since the helicopter was an old Mi-8, it needed to do a roller take-off; one which started from the dispersal itself between all our helicopters parked in the vicinity. What was most unusual was the amount the Mi-8 was made to roll just on its nose wheel. The result was a nearly collapsed nose oleo, which gave it a near-level attitude even when parked on the ground. If that wasn't enough, it flew with normal car batteries lying in the cargo compartment that were connected with a cable to the external power socket, that too outside the aircraft! The Congo was indeed a place that never ceased to amaze even the most experienced. Finally, after a few years, the Mi-8 crashed near Walikale; and it was the IAF that mounted the rescue operations.

### Sex Demo!

A lazy afternoon in February 2004 was hardly a befitting precursor to what was in store for us in the evening. A civilian lady doctor from MONUC, Dr Margaret Agama, was to deliver an awareness lecture on HIV/AIDS for all the personnel. This lady from Ghana looked like any other buxom local lady—only much more polished and well dressed. She spent the better part of an hour educating the uninitiated on the intricacies of the dreaded virus and its contraction, while the audience listened with rapt attention. It is very rare that one gets to see a woman completely at ease and totally in control in a hall full of 200 men who have been away from home for about seven months, lecturing them on safe-sex practices, with a condom in one hand and a smooth wooden replica of the male member in the other! The interactive talk was extremely effective, to say the least, though her poise and straightforward manner did cause some of our uninitiated brethren to squirm, blush, stare or show signs of all of the above-mentioned emotions—and then some more!

## An Armed Helicopter

The UN's bureaucratic framework is well known. Perhaps in a cauldron and cacophony of so many countries, differing views, opinions and national interests, this is an inevitable fall-out; otherwise, perceptions of bias, dominance and other prejudices would be predominant. A case in point was our pre-departure preparations at New Delhi. MONUC's requirement was for four attack helicopters (24x7, with year-round readiness) at two different detachment locations. Foreseeing the possible gaps in the future, I advised UN inspectors and officers to cater for Mi-17 weapon trusses so that it could serve as an armed helicopter and a back-up if needed. This was turned down by the UN on three counts: it was not part of the paperwork, i.e., MoU; MONUC aviation would never allow a Mi-17 in an armed role; and very importantly, no reimbursement was possible for this specialized equipment.

Anyway, my squadron, christened the IAF Squadron 2004, carried a set of trusses and rocket pods (free of charge!) just in case. One fine day in January 2004, a convoy of twenty-seven trucks of a humanitarian group under UN cover was ambushed and waylaid at Tubimbi, about 150 km south of Bukavu. Two Mi-25s were busy in Ituri providing fire support to a mission where a Milob had been shot, and anyway were almost a day away from the scene. One at

Goma was undergoing maintenance and would not be available for the next three days. As Murphy would have it, the only available Mi-25 had a major technical problem and would be down for at least a day. Under normal circumstances, this would not create any issue and operations would have been suitably delayed. However, these were not usual times; the convoy had reported sporadic fire and was in imminent danger with militias tactically deployed at vantage positions in the hills around.

No time could be lost, and MONUC and the Brigade HQ at Bukavu were desperate for solutions. Ground troops from Bukavu had refused to go by road without the fire cover of the Mi-25s. Overnight, with requisite clearances from Kinshasa, a Mi-17 was configured in the armed role with 192 rockets (57mm)—this made it look even more menacing and uglier than the Mi-25. It escorted the other three Mi-17s carrying fully armed troops into, literally, the heart of the matter. The militiamen simply vanished on seeing the armed-to-the-teeth helicopter doing dummy dives at them. Had they not run away, the clearance to fire was in hand. So much for the UN's bureaucratic foresight! This action helped MONUC demilitarize the two most insecure areas of Tubimbi and Kilungutwe, which were previously occupied by Rwandan Hutu rebels and Mayi-Mayi militiamen. UN reports officially logged that humanitarian aid was able to move into Tubimbi area after a full five years.

### Strange Bedfellows!

One afternoon in September 2003, a massacre was reported about 100 km from Bunia town in Ituri. This was to be one of the first robust responses by MONUC after taking over from the French-led stabilizing force earlier that year. Indian Mi-25s got ready for action, but Bangladeshi Mi-17s (recently inducted as Banair) expressed reservations, namely, about operating only on approved helipads and cruising speeds limited to 160 km/hr as per their LOA, or letter of assist (or how to avoid trouble!). The risky operation required a high-speed approach, dropping troops from low hover and, in general, a most flexible and adaptive mindset. To serve as role models, two Indian Mi-17s at Goma were forewarned of immediate deployment by the Force HQ at Kinshasa late at night. An early morning take-off with the sunrise allowed us to land at Bunia by 9 a.m. I led with Bhola and Pranay as apprentices, to learn about combat-flying first-hand.

Operations commenced (commando-style) with troops from the Pakistani brigade or PAKBATT taking part in two sets of low-hover drops to trap and apprehend the belligerents. Mi-25s provided fire cover and elaborate deception plans were suitably followed. The success of the mission became the talking point of the town and MONUC, very importantly, sent a loud message of what deterrence and retribution meant under Chapter VII of UN Military Action. Banair, too, got their act together and started to 'perform'.

It was only in the evening over drinks, and amid much mutual back-slapping, that I realized that the Pakistani troops belonged to none other than the Northern Light Infantry that had taken part in the Kargil War against India in 1999. Pervez Musharraf had sent them to a UN mission as a reward. Incidentally, I too had commanded a Mi-17 unit that had taken part in the same war (from the other side, of course). Truly, UN peacekeeping made strange bedfellows! Notwithstanding, South Asian cooperation and joint operations in the Congo bodes well for the future in terms of a unique peacekeeping model, provided the historical legacy can be sorted out first.

## Indian Jugaad

Our UN LOA for Mi-17 operations specified a radius of action (ROA) of 215 nautical miles. But, practically speaking, this was not possible. Internal tanks were prohibited by UN rules when carrying troops or passengers, so in all likelihood the stipulated ROA would leave one with no fuel at the end of the return trip, after discounting all other odds such as the quick-changing weather. Trust the UN bureaucracy (read Department of Field Support, or DFS) to make an issue out of it and insist on no leeway. The superlative performance, professionalism and courage that we had demonstrated, and of which the Department of Peace Keeping (DPKO) was in complete admiration, obviously had no effect on the DFS. Quite clearly, the chaps who had gone to New York to negotiate the LOA had goofed up.

Indian jugaad took over; this is a Hindi term meaning suitable adaptations incorporating copying, innovating and testing the limits of science and technology, etc.! My technical officer Ravi and I got on to some serious and survival-induced brainstorming. After a few trials and errors, and a whole lot of in-house welding, a trolley-tank stood fabricated. This was essentially a 900-litre auxiliary tank of the Mi-17 welded on to a wheeled ground trolley, along with the all-pervasive white paint and bold black 'UN' written across it. It passed UN muster with the inspectors gladly accepting it because it worked and was safe. We suspected that an additional overriding reason could have been that the UN (DFS) had incurred no extra cost! The idea was to carry two such tanks in one helicopter to a staging base; carry out operations, then refuel with the integral electric pump and return to base. Many mass area-domination sorties were enabled by this jugaad. Actually, as an unintended consequence, it increased the ROA by much more than 215 nm, and in turn the reach of MONUC. Subsequently, this mode of operation even increased the ROA of the Mi-25s with Mi-17 support.

### Combat Search and Rescue

Every year, 29 May is observed as the International Day of United Nations Peacekeepers—and we received information at 6 a.m. that some military observers or Milobs had been killed in Kalehe. Immediately, Pranay and I in a Mi-17, Gill and John in the attack chopper, and Sartaj with Pinto in another Mi-17 got airborne for the area. Gill and John set up a combat air patrol (CAP), which stopped the militia from firing at my Mi-17. On locating the crashed vehicle, I went in for landing in a very confined area full of elephant grass and next to high-tension cables. A dozen fully armed troops jumped out to take positions. They were received on the ground by a bloodstained Romanian Milob team leader, who explained that one Milob had died, while another, a lady, was missing. I stayed on the spot for a good twenty-five minutes with the cyclic control in my hands nearly at its rightmost extreme; all guns were pointing at the militia positions from where firing had been observed.

Overhead, meanwhile, Gill saw a group of rebels running towards the site. To deter them from targeting my helicopter, twenty-eight rockets were fired, which immediately dispersed them into the bushes. The medicos took the dead Milob on board, but since the lady could not be found, the team leader and armed troops elected to stay behind while I took off. While the militia were stopped from belligerence by counter-fire from the UN troops and the attack chopper, an RPG was fired as seen from the Mi-17 overhead (it missed and splashed in the lake).

Another nineteen troops were heli-inserted into Kalehe a little while later. My second shuttle was done without any top cover. However, the area had been sanitized by UN troops by then.

As plans were being made to lift the troops from Panji and insert them into Kalehe, news was received at 11 a.m. that the lady Milob had been located. Since the entire lot had come under threat from the rebels, the plan was changed and it was decided to extract all personnel immediately. However, 'immediately' in the UN takes several hours and the operation was launched only in the afternoon after necessary clearances.

The lady was evidently in a state of shock and had to be helped into the Mi-17. On landing in Goma, she told her story, which went thus. She and the deceased Milob had been following the team leader's Ford Four-Runner towards Bukavu when some militiamen stopped them. Deciding that it was an attempt to loot them, they decided to drive through. While doing so, the Ghanaian Navy Milob driving the second vehicle took a round from behind in his head and died on the spot. The vehicle went off road, hit a tree and turned turtle, upon which the Zambian lady Milob took cover in the tall grass. When she saw that the nearby village was deserted, she returned to the grass and hid till rescued.

## Walikale Wit

We got a taste of the hostile attitude and intentions of the Congolese militia again in July. I had gone for a sortie to Walikale with Sood, carrying a high-level UN delegation from New York. Fortunately, we were also carrying six South African troops as security and another four who were transiting. The sortie was uneventful till Walikale. After about one hour on ground, four Congolese army (ex-ANC) soldiers approached us and asked for written permission allowing the UN flight to land at Walikale. We shooed them away. They then went across half a kilometre and asked all the civilian delegates to show their passports. They further insisted that the flight would not be allowed to take-off unless permission was obtained. They were also not ready to see any reason and no amount of persuasion helped. A South African soldier (they all knew Swahili) guarding the Mi-17, quietly told me that rebel reinforcements were fifteen minutes away and we were nearing a hostage situation. Things could have got out of hand and turned nasty if not for some quick thinking.

Realizing that there were only two militiamen who were armed, I told all the UN and civil negotiators to get in the aircraft (actually, the engines were started and the high-level team, ladies included, left everything and ran back almost half a kilometre to the helicopter, displaying exemplary self-preservation skills!). I gave an ultimatum to the Congolese militia leader that the helicopter was taking off and if they tried to obstruct it, they could expect debilitating return fire. Seeing themselves outnumbered and outgunned, the Congolese relented and backed off. As the helicopter took off, two trucks filled with fully armed militiamen could be seen speeding towards the helipad. South African troops had the ability to be intuitive and perceptive about militia behaviour. It comes from their legacy—they are mostly an amalgamation of different militia groups after the apartheid regime went out.

## Human Trafficking and Sex Abuse

Rape has been used extensively as a weapon of war by virtually all the forces involved in the Congo conflict. Soldiers and rebel fighters have engaged in acts of sexual violence to attack the fundamental values of a community, to scare the civilian population into submission, to punish them for allegedly supporting enemy forces or to provide gratification for the fighters. Thousands of women have also been abducted and kept as slaves in camps to provide sexual, domestic and agricultural services. Often, combatants took the women's clothes so that they could not run away. We once did a mission to one such village—quickly abandoned on arrival of our

Mi-25. MONUC estimated at least 25,000 cases of sexual violence a year in North Kivu province alone. In early 2006, Mayi-Mayi groups were reported to have raped countless women and children in Katanga province. Men and boys in increasing numbers were also not spared sexual assault.

The majority of uniformed personnel and civilian contractors working in peacekeeping operations do so honourably. They risk their lives to repair the damage and destruction of war. Tragically, however, international organizations and activists have documented a disturbing link with these deployments—and sometimes within themselves too. One observation was that, in and around the same regions where one finds established, long-term international deployments, one also sees a dramatic rise in the number of trafficked women and girls. Members of the MONUC peacekeeping force did commit abuses against displaced women and girls. The highly publicized scandal over UN peacekeepers and child prostitution led to an investigation by the UN Office of Internal Oversight Services. The office identified a pattern of sexual exploitation by uniformed personnel involving women and girls and asked the concerned troop-contributing countries to take swift disciplinary action.

A similar pattern was seen in the Balkans. Sex trafficking is more than just prostitution; it is about people being sold, being denied their passports and being forced to pay off bogus debts to their traffickers. It is also about organized crime and, in post-conflict regions, a transnational threat. Most organizations that work to combat human trafficking have devoted considerable resources to assisting and rehabilitating victims, documenting the phenomenon, advocating legislative changes, attempting to create witness protection programmes and prosecuting traffickers. Hats off to these committed Good Samaritans.

Human trafficking, like other forms of organized crime, shapes the security environment of post-conflict regions. Some uniformed service members, civilian contractors and civil servants tend to deny links between trafficking and peacekeeping deployments; they fail to understand the security implications of both human rights abuses and the unwitting support of organized crime. How leadership and officers understand trafficking affects how they will implement policy. The degree to which government officials take any issue seriously always determines what they are willing to do about it and what resources—people, money and time—they are willing to devote to it.

Our contingents in the Congo had a very clean record on this front. Understandably, it was easier to achieve this state, unlike most infantry units, because of the insulation provided by the confined and secured nature of aviation camps. As leaders, we had zero tolerance on this account. Repatriation and retribution were assured in proven cases. A strict one-year term only ensured a better understanding of all social and operational issues but did not let complacency and fatigue set in. All personnel were sent home twice in a year's stint. Leading from the front meant the first sets of dos and don'ts were applied to leaders before others. This, singularly perhaps, was the most important step.

In our camp, we had regular reiteration of moral values, danger of diseases and the responsibility to loved ones at home. Potential 'loose' cases, sometimes easily identifiable, were given extra attention by supervising officers. Interaction with the general public was limited to strictly regulated 'hearts and minds' campaigns. A concerted effort was made right from pre-deployment days to aim for a home-away-from-home. All facilities for sports, recreation, education, Bollywood films, cable TV and even a sauna bath had been catered for and set up as a priority. A point being missed out by many militaries was that a fall in core values such as morality, discipline, ethics, among others, would not be left behind in the Congo; it would go back to the home country and result in further degradation of soldier-like qualities. This is a crucial issue for armies that are professional and mean business in the future.

### Don't Cry for Me

The Democratic Republic of the Congo has borne the worst of colonialism: a past whose darkness is so candidly brought out in researched works like *King Leopold's Ghost*, with a conservative death toll of 10 million in just twenty-three years (1885–1908) and a present that continues to batter poverty-stricken Congolese with every criminal act and horrific method known to man. The daily death toll due to malnutrition and lack of healthcare because of the strife is around 1,500.

Even when the Belgians left, it is widely believed that the US and the ex-colonists of the Congo ensured that the first elected president (Lumumba) was assassinated and replaced by an inept, corrupt but compliant General Mobutu—in a way, the 'whites' never left.* Once, while flying in an area that was reputed to be close to the mines that supplied uranium for the two atomic bombs of Hiroshima and Nagasaki, a Congolese UN worker spoke of a legend—the US Marines still guarded the mines. One will never know the truth, since the area was out of bounds. But it is a fact that unscrupulous businesses and multinationals from the West, and now China, pull the real strings. Various players in the fray for exploiting the mineral wealth do what they do to feed insatiable appetites. Even under the rubric of peacebuilding, and right under the nose of the World

* Susan Williams, *White Malice: The CIA and the Covert Recolonization of Africa* (New York: PublicAffairs, 2021).

Bank, the Congolese government sold off the rights of 75 per cent of the copper and cobalt reserves in a shady deal that reportedly brought no gains to the state or the people.

Slavery in illegal mines, sexual exploitation and abuse, crimes against children, etc., are all there to be seen in the Congo even today. It seems that the 2006 elections just managed to transfer the tools of power and exploitation from one set of hands to another. Whether real sustainable peace is even possible in the current format of peacebuilding, whose terms are driven by the donor community, only time will tell. Africa, and in particular the Congo, requires India's help, but in the current UNPK context where we are only contributing troops, the results are highly debatable. The large Indian diaspora in eastern Congo told us many times that India can really help, provided the West allows us to! We definitely should not end up doing someone's dirty work; even if they proclaim us to be the gold standard in peacekeeping. Joseph Conrad's *Heart of Darkness* surely has an underlying message that the real darkness lies elsewhere, in the greed of man, especially in those that have been causing Africa to bleed for centuries.

# TOUCHING ALL CORNERS

# PURABI PRAKASH

THIS TITLE TRANSLATES as 'the eastern light', and is quite apt since the Seven Sisters, or the seven north-eastern states, as they are sometimes collectively called, witness the first sunrise in India every day. Back in the 1980s, life was hard as a military aviator with constant deployments in exotic locales across these states and also Bhutan. It was a cultural contrast too, with people and their lives personifying simplicity, music and community care.

The stories here are about pilots operating in a challenging and hazardous environment, especially during the prolonged monsoons. Chopper pilots have helped in road-building in the mountains, carried famous politicians and other leaders with their own quirks and whims across the region, saved lives and, at the same time, operated against militants. They offer unique glimpses of this region such as the 'happiness' in Bhutan and many others.

## Hashi Hustle

After training at the Helicopter Training School (HTS) as a newly commissioned pilot officer, I was posted to Hashimara along with my coursemate Kots. He was actually a course senior, but he did his helicopter conversion with me. We made our rail reservations together for a long but memorable journey. Those were the times of normal postal service, where joining instructions reached so late that one got it as a redirected post at the new station. So we were unprepared for what followed. Kots' parents had come from Bombay (before it became Mumbai) to see him off at Secunderabad railway station. After the usual pleasantries with his parents, I moved away to allow them a few private moments. Looking inside our first-class cabin, I saw a beautiful young girl sitting there. I was overjoyed—and I could not wait to share the news with Kots. But he was busy with his parents. I managed to pull him away for a minute and told him. We went over to the window and he looked in, and, with a straight face, but I suspect fully enjoying the moment, he said, 'There is just one problem—she is my sister who has come to see me off.' I just about managed to make him promise that he would not let it out to his family. Many years later, we served together again at Hyderabad where his sister, now married with kids, met my wife and shared this story.

It was a three-night train journey with two changeovers at Calcutta (now Kolkata) and Jalpaiguri. From Jalpaiguri, the rail tracks changed to metre-gauge and a slower but quaint train. We went into the foothills to cross River Teesta and passed many lush tea gardens. At one time, the train came to an abrupt halt. An elephant herd was crossing the tracks, and taking its time to do so. We remained on the lookout since we were in Jaldapara National Park.

By the time we reached Hashimara, it was midnight and pitch-dark because of the usual electricity outage. Also, it was pouring cats and dogs. The station master was going around with a lantern, shouting 'Hashimara'. This is exactly how it is described in the joining instructions with a touch of humour. But, as I said, that reached us after a few weeks of arrival, redirected from Hyderabad. The only mode of travel was the rickshaw and somehow, we got two of them to agree to ferry us to the airbase. However, the station master would not allow us to go, assuring us of sure robbery or even worse on the way. A group of twenty cyclists intervened and agreed to escort us. They turned out to be airmen from the base who had come to see off one of their colleagues. They confirmed that the worries of the station master were bang on and not misplaced.

## Squadron Life in Hashi

Kots and I shared a room—and obviously one toilet and bath. It was painful since both of us were late risers and had to report for early morning briefings together. After a few months, we ensured that at least one of us was out on detachment at Aizawl or other places. Any rare weekend together meant borrowing a mobike and speeding off to Phuntsholing in Bhutan to do what bachelors normally do! The place was also good for foreign smuggled goods, such as electronic gadgets, which we so desired at that point of time. Life was simple—happiness was even simpler and cheaper to get. Coming back to Hashi by night on a single bike was suicidal—encounters with gangs of robbers were frequent. So, officers used to tie up beforehand to come back in a group—honking away merrily.

Times were changing. Bharti, a shares–debentures-savvy brother officer—a rare variety—got a Maruti 800 from the first-ever lot produced. It was a star attraction, especially given its mileage. So was Guru's Ind-Suzuki motorcycle, which gave a mileage of forty-odd kilometres. However, the downsides were revealed in a freak hailstorm with hailstones as big as cricket balls coming down. A Kal Baisakhi (a very powerful thunderstorm) had hit us in the evening and there were many injuries. But the main insult was the large pockmarks on the Maruti and the complete destruction of the Ind-Suzuki's fuel tank. Fiat and Ambassador owners had a good laugh, but not for too long I am afraid, as the years passed. Kots and I had bicycles since we had still not saved up enough to buy motorcycles.

Fighter aircraft such as Hunters gave way to MiG-21 squadrons. We had a volleyball court in the middle of the base, where passionate battles between squadrons and other groupings used to take place. At stake was paying for the endless plates of pakoras at the end. The colour and fervour of the verbal exchanges far exceeded the skills displayed in the do-or-die matches. There was a single music system to enliven the whole process, and it belonged to Zapo—our most mentally evolved colleague. He later rose to be my AOC-in-C at Central Air Command.

Bachelors would 'bounce', akin to a forced call-on, couples at their homes for late-night binges on weekends. To reciprocate, we would organize large bonfire parties at the mess at least once a month. It was an important element of bonding, which today has been lost, as have many other useful social niceties. Home theatres, the internet and mobiles are slowly eating away at the time and space we had for others. This is something to think about for people who will do combat together. While station camaraderie rarely used to go beyond the guardroom when you left on posting, you always had your buddy's back. Today, WhatsApp is ensuring you are never out of virtual touch, but completely out of 'real' touch!

## Pate (Tummy)-Puja

The most vibrant place in a squadron is the cafeteria with its attached kitchen that can cater to any unique taste, and, at the same time, produce such standardized taste that no chef can dare copy. A legacy of our officers' messes is the number of egg preparations. Let the English have their scrambled or sunny side up, IAF pilots can beat everyone hands down in variety. An example is ande ki bhujia (a cousin of scrambled eggs, shall we say). There is the 'sookha' or dry variety, which is the closest cousin. And then there are the 'dheela' (loose), 'geela' (wet) and more than a dozen other kinds in between. Then come the toppings on the single- or double-fried egg—varying from 'kadak' (full of chillies) to mixes that will beat varieties offered by Domino's Pizza!

Once upon a time, when free rations had just come in, our officers' messes achieved a standardization that would have been envied in flying standard operating procedures. All across India, tea was of the same taste—and unpalatable. It emerged later that the contractor of the army supply corps was the same whose tender bid had been the lowest. As pay commissions passed and incomes increased, this improved, and today's youngsters can be grateful for a good cup of tea in the morning.

Then there are the varieties of eaters. Vegetarianism was not in vogue thirty years back, but there were enough other types. Besides the rock-solid vegetarian, there was the Bengali vegetarian—someone who considered fish a vegetarian delicacy. In fact, they even called it 'Jal-Tori', 'tori' being a vegetable and 'jal' being water. Then there was the eggetarian who was okay with eggs but no further. Those were financially frugal times and the hardly affordable chicken was a prized dish at parties—and always less in quantity. This produced a 'mokatarian' type; 'moka' is opportunity in Hindi—one who would have chicken outside but not serve it in his vegetarian home!

## Boozy Tales

While the Western tradition of gulping drinks once in a while suits that climate, we Indians tend to hit the bottle only in the evening. Back in the northeast at that time, there was literally nothing else to do. Doordarshan had only news or classical stuff and the odd episode of *Chitrahaar* that played Bollywood songs, which we looked forward to. So it was that even a teetotaller took to a drink or two to lower his inhibitions in the bar. Rum was preferred and the macho choice. Some others preferred whisky. I remember Mulla Feroze in Hashi who preferred whisky when offered but served us Apsoo (rum) when we bounced at his house. It was an infamous brand that only the strongest palate could withstand—also, it was the cheapest. Bar closing time was indicated by barmen asking for last drinks. There were some interesting drinkers like 'Toddy' who used to line up six drinks as his last ones and promptly go off to sleep after the first. The balance drinks were picked up by thirsty bachelors like me, followed by picking up and dropping Toddy to his room. I have always wondered if he did it on purpose to humour us.

### Weekend Binges

Those days, weekends started on Saturdays, around 2 p.m. after work. More often than not, one would find the entire station, from the air officer commanding (AOC) to all COs and others, in the bar for a customary beer. After the bosses would leave, some argument or the other would crop up with everyone taking sides—and more beer and pakoras would flow. Closer to 5 p.m., the entire lot would move to the volleyball court to decide the argument—since verbal debates inevitably failed. The hard-fought duels on the volleyball court would lead to the losers funding the evening binge. Couples staying far away would also join in and merry-making would continue till late into the night. No wonder most of the first half of Sundays were spent sleeping.

## Northeast Nation-Building

In a TV advertisement for tourism, a little-known fact sprang up—the Ahom dynasty in Assam was the only one that no one could subdue, not even the mighty Mughals. Those of us who have served in the Northeast will acknowledge the indomitable spirit and resilience of the people. The strong sense of identity and other causes have thrown up a series of insurgency movements across all the seven states since Independence. The Indian armed forces have been involved in putting down or controlling these fires over the decades, starting with the Naga problem. IAF helicopters have played a crucial part in supporting the Indian Army in counter-insurgency strategies in Nagaland, Mizoram (the most successful campaign), Tripura, Assam, and even Meghalaya and Arunachal.

The biggest issue in countering insurgency is the inevitable lack of boots-on-ground. This is where medium-lift helicopters of the IAF have pitched in over the decades, mobilizing troops from one place to another; in short, acting as enablers and force multipliers. Where required, they have been used in the offensive support role such as against the ULFA across in Bhutan. Counter-insurgency is only a part of the strategy to integrate the Northeast with the mainland. The other more important part is holistic development and nation-building activities; choppers have played an equally important role in that too.

## Border Buniyaad

A major reason for carrying out air operations anywhere in the world is because of non-connectivity by road. The Border Roads Organisation, or BRO, along with the engineers of the army, are responsible for building roads in border areas, which help speedy deployment during war. The BRO is doing yeoman service in building infrastructure all across the seven states. Helicopters play a critical part in reconnaissance, conveying of workers and officers, airlifting supplies that cannot reach there by any other means, and in many other ways. The Mi-17 is a versatile machine, capable of carrying loads inside as well as outside. This capability of the aircraft has been exploited by many forces in the world. Bulldozers of the BRO that can cut through mountains too have an admirable record and weigh more than a Mi-17. Alas, even the multifaceted Mi-17 has its limits. A partnership between the BRO and the IAF station at Mohanbari was possible, and it was pioneered as a revolutionary concept in 1999.

The time was ripe for the Siachen Tigers, which I was commanding, to come to the fore. Considerable planning and meticulous study of Mi-17 charts and manuals, as also geography and topography, resulted in a unique plan. Bulldozers were dismantled into smaller parts to get them within limits of the aircraft's capability. Missions were envisioned and planned to the remotest of helipads in the most treacherous terrain, some even without helipads. The objective was to trek on ground (aircrew included), along the proposed road axis and select suitable areas as future helipads. Some of these were never-ventured-into areas. Thereafter, a helicopter would drop or winch in equipment so that a rough clearing could be made.

A basic clearing allowed Mi-17s to under-sling bulldozers (in manageable pieces) since landing was impossible. This included cumbersome gantries (chains and pulleys) that allowed heavy equipment to be assembled manually, and also fuel and rations. The bulldozer would then carve out a helipad and regular supply of equipment, rations and personnel could begin. Theoretically speaking, each such helipad would allow two additional road-building avenues along the mountain slopes. Thus, three such helipads on the Chakla Gaon axis in Arunachal cut down the road-building time to one-sixth. Such sorties are extremely demanding and test the limits of the performance envelope of Mi-17 helicopters. Similar activities have been supported by IAF helicopters in building dams, bridges, hydel plants, advance landing grounds and many others. A total of twenty-four bulldozers, four trucks, one roadroller and nine heavy air compressors were airlifted in an effort to link these inaccessible regions by road in the first year itself. The then chief minister wrote to the air chief in glowing terms of this feat in 2002. Nothing is impossible with helicopters; it just takes a little time!

The most visible role, and also the most satisfying for pilots, is saving lives and humanitarian assistance. An unknown fact is that IAF helicopters all over the Northeast are always on standby to assist civilians in medical evacuation, e.g., to deal with epidemics. Disasters such as the Arunachal flash floods in 2000, the Sikkim earthquake in 2012 and perennial floods in Assam have showcased IAF helicopters giving their professional best in support of citizens. Thousands of medical evacuations all over the Northeast over the last four decades are a legacy that is part of the story of integrating and developing the 'seven sisters'.

## Just Another Day(s)

That helicopter pilots by necessity need to be multiskilled and adaptable is a truism demonstrated on a daily basis across the country. What better example than the one on 1 November 1999. I, along with a just-posted-in flying officer, was airborne at sunrise from Tawang, at a 10,000-foot altitude, for the super-cyclone relief in Odisha in our Mi-17. Bad weather was encountered abeam Tezpur, forcing us to land there and wait. By about 7.30 a.m., HQ Eastern Air Command sent a message tasking us with a most unusual requirement. A MiG-21 crash a few days back had thrown up a unique challenge. The engine, the prime suspect of the crash, had to be retrieved to be investigated for faulty maintenance by the foreign manufacturer and warranty invocation.

However, it was located in the densely forested Kaziranga sanctuary, half-buried in a completely inaccessible ravine. A plan was made and I, along with an engineering officer and few air warriors, were winched down by a Chetak close to the site. After a tough trek, we reached the site. Some useful out-of-the-box thinking and innovative suggestions by the youngsters allowed the engine to be semi-dug out and wrapped with steel cables (from the transport section). A few hours later, we approached the site in our Mi-17 and executed an out-of-ground effect, or OGE hover, since we could not come lower than 30 metres due to the tall trees. Very unconventionally, three sets of 10-metre cables were joined, and the engine was virtually prised out of the ground by the powerful Mi-17. It was dropped on to a vehicle about 5 km ahead at the nearest kutcha track. By the time we landed in Tezpur, it was sunset. After a well-deserved rest, we reached Bhubaneswar by afternoon the next day. Two days of flood relief later, we were tasked with a winch retrieval of a Pilotless Target Aircraft (PTA) from the deep sea—a demanding task itself. So there it was—from high-altitude air maintenance to unconventional under-slung to flood relief in inclement weather to PTA retrieval by winching. While I was an experienced pilot, it must have been a great learning experience for the young flying officer on his first operational stint. Such are the business-as-usual demands on a helicopter pilot!

**Lohit Leela**

The beautiful Lohit Valley in the far-eastern corner of India straddles the River Lohit. It was only in 2004 that the valley was properly bridged with the floodplains and towns of Tezu and Chowkham. The main bridge at the mouth of the valley lies at a famed shrine of Parsuram Kund. Tezu has an airstrip that was extensively used during the 'over the hump' operations of WWII. It was also the point where we ended our twin trekking expedition to Chakla Gaon and the tri-junction boundary point between India, China and Myanmar. This was flagged in by the chief minister of Arunachal Pradesh in

2001 with the entire population of Tezu in attendance. Among the guests of honour were 'gaon-budhas', or village elders, from the Mishmi and other tribes across the valley.

Hayuliang, which lies just inside the hills, has many roads branching out to the valleys of Chakla Gaon and Walong, among others. It was our base for launching winching sorties by the hundreds for the BRO, allowing roads to be built that are strategic in nature. The valleys were too narrow for the larger Mi-26s, so dozers and other heavy earth movers were broken down to be carried by our Mi-17s. Along the eastern-most road, further upstream, lies the hamlet of Walong. It is an important army post and advanced landing ground, as also a site for the famous Battle of Walong during the 1962 war with China. Many Mi-4 sorties were done from here to evacuate and reinforce the Indian Army during that war. Along with the battle for Rezang La in Ladakh, Walong shares the honour of display of courage and tenacity of the highest order by our soldiers. In 2004, a beautiful memorial was inaugurated as a tribute to them. The valley was maintained by IAF Caribous and Otters for decades. A Caribou airframe is part of the war memorial. As a pilot officer in 1983–84, I flew a number of sorties as a passenger to Walong in both these aircraft, while stationed at Guwahati and Chabua. The highest skill level of seat-of-pants flying were amply on display. I distinctly remember Srikant, a Caribou pilot, who had handled up to ten single-engine emergencies and one both-engine failure. It was a fantastic aeroplane with flaps all across its straight wings that allowed it to climb out from ALGs like a chopper—vertically.

Before the main war memorial came up in 2004, there was a smaller one at the site. While commanding the Siachen Tigers, I had observed that this memorial kept getting inaugurated by various senior dignitaries of the armed forces, each time with a traditional plaque-laying ceremony. The unit's CO had a simple explanation—

after fifteen days, they would simply remove it, throw it into the Lohit and await the next VIP. His motto: 'All's well when every VIP feels good!'

We (Siachen Tigers) started our tri-junction trek from a point ahead of Kibithu. Our close association with the then stationed Gurkha battalion helped since they provided two soldiers as guides. The unit was commanded by Colonel Bipin Rawat, who later headed the Indian Army and became the country's first chief of defence staff. The association was an exemplary display of jointmanship. During the trek, we discovered the wreckage of a WWII USAF bomber. This report led to, in later years, a massive search for other such remnants across Arunachal. Many families back in the USA got a sense of closure after more than half a century.

One memorable story involved carrying an army mule from Kibithu to Gompa just across the Lohit. This was a special mule, a 'Mule MA', which is able to carry heavier barrels or mortar pieces. MA stands for mountain artillery while others are GS or general service. Mules are a cross between a male donkey and a mare. They are intelligent and hardy but very stubborn. After initial detailed planning of crating and sedation, the sortie materialized one fine morning. I had a revolver just in case the animal went berserk. The duration was only fifteen to twenty minutes, so we were not really worried—reassured by the strong wooden crate and heavy sedation. All went well till we were airborne. Then all hell broke loose with the animal thrashing around wildly with its famous rear-leg kicks. My gunner was updating me with the happenings—the hapless mule drivers were trying to control the animal and save themselves at the same time. The mule settled down just before landing, once it had completely shattered the wooden crate. To our good luck, nothing else was damaged and no one was seriously hurt.

## Golfing Paradise

Upper Assam boasts the highest concentration of golf courses in the world, perhaps only behind some areas of Switzerland. Every tea garden has a course complete with a club house and all ancillaries that go with the tradition of golf. The unique Assam 'ghas', or grass, is short and stubby, requiring no maintenance except grazing by the equally short and stubby Assamese cattle. Greens are, of course, protected by barbed wire. Each club holds its own mega whole-weekend event annually. Ladies compete with each other over the best food laid out and dances are organized. Gents or managers chill over beer and a round of golf. It is a hard life for the managers at their estates, which belie their palatial bungalows. Workers' unions and unrest are common and require experience and deftness in handling. My NDA coursemate was a manager in one of the estates and I became well-versed with all their nuances. It was risky too—with ULFA, SULFA and other extortionists abounding during the 1990s. I remember the unfortunate fatal lynching of Mandher, a Khalsa tea estate manager, by his workers over some trivial issue. His daughter was studying at the same boarding school as my daughter—Welham in Dehradun.

The culminating golf event in winters was the Assam Open. Everyone landed up for it, including well-known amateur champions from across the country. The two-day event involved a number of functions and merry-making. Air Marshal 'Raja' from the command headquarters had decided to come and play in one such event. But he left after playing just three holes. The story went thus. Back at the home course in Shillong, Raja's regular caddy used to place the ball after every shot as a proverbial 'lollipop'. It is said in the armed forces' golfing circuit that a general never 'loses his ball' or is never out of bounds. However, back at Digboi in the Assam

Open, Raja was not allowed his regular caddy—and there were no lollipops. After three disastrous holes, the air marshal retired hurt—in every way!

## Rafting the Siang

The Brahmaputra is the greatest landmark of north-east India. Wide as a large lake during floods, it is the soul of Assam. While tributaries such as the Lohit and Subansiri are iconic in themselves, it is the mighty Siang, known as the Tsang-Po in China, which is the heart of the Brahmaputra. In terms of volume and flow, it is unmatched in India.

Earlier, Arunachal was mostly closed to foreign tourists and only a sprinkling of Indians visited, mostly the famed monastery at Tawang. However, as part of opening up Arunachal to all, a number of expeditions were planned in the early 1990s. One such Indo-US rafting expedition was planned in December 1992. The river had never been rafted across its turbulent length till the town of Pasighat in the foothills. Among professional rafters in the US, it was rated just below the Yellow River in China, which is a known killer. Most of the team was American, including some of the best guides and experts and some rich tourists who had funded the expedition. There were six IAF officers led by me with good experience on most Indian rivers. There were four 18-foot rafts in all; however, either by design or default, ours (Indian team) ended up being the heaviest with the most load in it besides the six of us. The IAF got involved through two organizers who were ex-air marshals—MM and Sikki. For some strange reason, there was a clear dividing line between the two sides, at least initially. Later, as days and episodes progressed, we got closer to the American tourists who were great people. The real problems were the organizers on both sides.

The starting point was Tuting, because further upstream was too dangerous. It had an advanced landing ground—a short grassy runway. The Americans were amazed that IAF An-32s carried out regular sorties on this stretch. And just to drive home the point, there was the wreckage of a crashed An-32 at one end. There were a total of seven camp sites en route—as also seven major rapids that counted as class four or five in terms of difficulty. Because of our heavier raft, we flipped over in five of them. The recovery part takes up to an hour, after a kilometre of bobbing up and down in the rapids with only the life jacket as a buoy. After we complained about the weight on our fourth flip, an American lady—a good fifty-plus in age—volunteered to be with us. After our subsequent and last flip, we climbed on board the up-turned raft collecting our mates. But the lady was nowhere in sight. As the rapids ended after half a kilometre, desperate attempts were made to locate her by the other three rafts and kayakers. As we readied for the drill to upright our own raft, I heard a feeble cry from below. She was trapped under our raft with an air bubble to support her. One of the expert kayakers came and prised her away safely, much to everyone's relief.

A big cultural event was organized at the midway town of Yingkiong. Arunachal's rich tribal diversity and legacy were on full display. The biggest hurdle came the next day—a rapid so ferocious and long that it took our breath away. After two hours of deliberation, it was decided that the tourists would walk the stretch on the narrow riverbanks. Most experts preferred portage, which meant physically picking up all the rafts and walking, avoiding the rapids altogether. In the end, Ron—the oldest guide and CEO of the US rafting company principally involved—single-handedly took a raft and went through, showing us the way. All of us followed with our hearts in our mouths—and surprisingly, we did not flip this time. At Pasighat, the whole town was there to greet us with great merriment. After due celebrations, we flew off the next day in IAF choppers to the airbase at Chabua. An evening was planned by 'Dushman', as our C-in-C was fondly referred to. The base was commanded by Ajax who had been my boss earlier in Jaisalmer. The six of us were made to retire early while the party continued. Our American friends were quite perplexed at these protocols—and we could not offer any logical explanations when we bid them goodbye in the morning.

## Piloting Politicians

The first time I came across Rajiv Gandhi was in 1984, when he had just been plucked out from being an airline pilot and placed into the hot seat of Indian politics. This was after the untimely demise of his younger brother, Sanjay Gandhi, who was deep into politics and had been the Congress heir apparent. Rajiv had just been appointed a secretary in the party, and his first political rally was at Kolasib, which was midway between Aizawl and Silchar. We flew him in our Chetak from Aizawl to Kolasib and back. He came across as a very likeable and handsome man who was clearly in an uncomfortable spot as compared to his pilot's seat. His speech was also unlike a hardened politician—the dramatics and rhetoric were missing. But his aura of vulnerability and naivety endeared him to the public at large. The rest, of course, is history.

Brigadier Sailo was the chief minister of Mizoram before the peace accord was signed in 1986. We flew him extensively all across the hundreds of helipads in the state. The standard routine was a lunch with the community at large, for which he became very popular. He forced us to accompany him as his special guests. This did allow us to have a ringside view of the subtle diversities within Mizo culture. The lunch would include various meats—some palatable, some not suited to our north Indian stomachs. Bamboo-shoot dishes were a certainty, and I developed a taste for them.

The diet was protein-rich and very healthy, with only traces of cooking oil. Brig. Sailo told me the interesting fact of a once-in-a-blue-moon flowering of the bamboo, and the famine that follows because of rats that multiply exponentially.

Lal Thanwala took over as the Congress chief minister of Mizoram after the elections in 1984. He was a good friend and very close to all IAF pilots—once again by virtue of helicopters being his only means to cover the hilly state. He was very fond of playing cards (bridge), which was one vice that I never managed to pick up. It was interesting to listen to him about how the insurgency and MNF (Mizo National Front) came about. According to him, the IAF's strafing of Aizawl in the 1960s actually jump-started the movement, giving it a new high. A very clear understanding of a mix of politics, ideology, corruption and crime, which encourages such movements to thrive, was apparent from the interactions with people in the thick of things. Counter-insurgency campaigns are far more complex and puzzling than a war campaign.

In Arunachal Pradesh, initial politics revolved only around Gegong Apang, after statehood was attained in 1986. He was a larger-than-life character who needs an entire book to cover all his colours and hues. His mainstay of covering the entire mountainous state was IAF helicopters. He was especially fond of moving around with his coterie in a Mi-17, which he trusted and relied upon completely. In turn, he was very magnanimous to the demands of the IAF in general and chopper squadrons in particular. Quite often he was dropped at various valleys in prominent towns and large villages to spend weekends. Legend has it that he had a wife and family in each one. Also, he behaved like an emperor. Siganporia, a Chetak squadron CO, dropped him at Itanagar at a wrongly designated helipad while the public was waiting at another. Despite Apang's protests and some harsh language in the local dialect, a professional Sigan did not relent. On getting down, both pilots were put under arrest. Only timely intervention by the Central government saved Sigan and his co-pilot from spending a night in jail.

It was, therefore, a welcome change to see subsequent rational chief ministers. When I was a CO in Mohanbari, I interacted a lot with Mukut Mithi, who later became a Rajya Sabha member. Our first meeting was during the flash floods of 2000. He was at Pasighat when the search for a doomed boat carrying more than a hundred people was on. After the dramatic rescue of all, he hugged us affectionately and we became his favourites. Tourism and hydel infrastructure were his top priorities. The IAF played a great part in both these sectors. He would always seek our advice when it came to building the aviation infrastructure in the state. This was the genesis of a large subsequent project that upgraded aviation infra at Tawang, Along, Menchuka, Anini, Pasighat and Walong. It was a big surprise one day when he and his friends landed up at my house in Shillong. I was just a wing commander posted there, but I was in Delhi then on temporary duty. He had come for a North Eastern Council (NEC) meeting. Everyone was taken by surprise, including my wife and my commander-in-chief. But that is the way he was—large-hearted and down to earth.

During the aftermath of the 2000 flash floods, a number of dignitaries came down to assess the damage and fiscal relief due. One remarkable politician that I flew around for three days was Nitish Kumar, who was then the Union minister of agriculture. His quiet and reticent manner and good powers of analysis were quite evident as he went through various presentations and meetings. He was very appreciative of our role in the rescue and rehab, and he ensured that the word reached Delhi. Later, as the chief minister, he turned Bihar around from the culture of lawlessness that it had mired itself in. There is a story that a Pakistani delegation wanted to study his work. Their logic—if Bihar could turn around, Pakistan could hope to do the same!

In 2001, Deputy Prime Minister L.K. Advani came for the inaugural 'Sindhu Darshan' on the banks of the Brahmaputra at Tezu. This was to be followed by a main festival in Leh, by the Indus. At that point in time, he exuded great inner strength and resolve. One can understand how painstakingly he put the Bharatiya Janata Party (BJP) on its future growth trajectory. A more memorable trip was to fly former defence minister George Fernandes in 2000 for seven days and touch all capitals of the Northeast states. This also included a night stay with the Indian Army at Tawang on Christmas Eve. For some inexplicable reason, he had decided that I was a Christian, and he profusely apologized the next day for keeping me away from my family during midnight mass. During this period, we got a free ringside view of the extremely rich and diverse tribal culture of the Northeast. In fact, at Kohima, Fernandes inaugurated the first Hornbill festival, which today is an extremely popular annual feature on the tourism map. At the end of seven days, before he got into the An-32 for Delhi, he insisted on spending half an hour in the crew room of the Siachen Tigers. It is an honour cherished till date by the squadron.

## Assam Courier—A Great Equalizer

The early 1980s were times that cannot be easily visualized today—connectivity was poor by road and rail, and virtually non-existent by air. Insurgency was at its peak with armed forces deployed all across the Northeast. A single ray of hope was a weekly Assam Courier from Bagdogra in An-12s. While the official capacity or green list was of bona fide passengers from various official quotas, the yellow list was of prime interest to the hundreds waiting. This was based on the captain's discretion, which involved various factors such as his skill, experience, confidence, mood and general benevolence. Things were not very organized in those days, nor was security such an issue. So, the yellow list number was decided by the captain (normally a white-bearded, wizened Khalsa) while walking to the An-12. A line of officers and enlisted men stood in a line (barely controlled or discernible). Quite obviously, the demand-supply gap was huge, and after the first few entrants—all hell broke loose. Rank and order went out of the window, and it was every man for himself (with his suitcase). The yellow list numbers were sacrosanct and gates promptly closed after that. There's a world of difference in today's Assam Courier—clockwork efficiency, first-rate infrastructure, air-conditioned waiting rooms and high security, among other civil airport atmospherics.

## Happiness: A Way of Life

Bhutan is one of the happiest countries in the world—long ago, its government declared that the 'happiness quotient' of the people was a more important issue than its gross domestic product (GDP)! I don't know about now, but when I operated for three years from Hashimara, between 1983 and 1986, it was certainly true. As I've mentioned in a story earlier, we used to regularly fly the royal family, except the king. His astrologer had prohibited him from flying in a single-engine chopper. Society at large was laid-back, content and devoted to their king. I saw a very interesting ceremony once, albeit from afar and a little discreetly. The IAF had an air traffic control detachment at Paro that used to handle just one aeroplane of Druk Air once in a blue moon. It was an annual ceremony involving a family bath. A large pit was dug next to the river Paro Chhu. A huge fire burned alongside, heating up large, round river stones. An entire family of at least four generations waited in the cold patiently. Then the men, with the help of large sticks, pushed the stones into the pit; at the same time, a channel of the river was opened from upstream. In the sizzling water, the entire family packed into the pit sans any clothes.

I heard a story about how devout Buddhist villagers were. Even though they were non-vegetarians, they would not kill their goats or yaks themselves for meat, especially before a village feast. They would trudge up a mountain with the animal. And from these heights they would facilitate the animal's fatal fall. I never managed to muster the courage to ask how!

A very big and welcome surprise awaited me in Hashimara one day. Phuntsholing in Bhutan, just on the border, was our favourite weekend spot. The only worthwhile hotel was Druk—a four-star. It was too expensive for us. One day, the manager of Druk called up the airbase on the landline (that was the only telephone) to leave a message for me that I was invited for dinner on Saturday. I was surprised since I didn't remember entering any lucky draw or other such scheme. I reached there on my bike to be greeted and escorted to a reserved table. And after a few minutes, the VIP who had invited me joined. It was my dad! He was the chief of protocol in the foreign ministry in Delhi and had come for a meeting to Thimpu. He had decided to surprise me on the way—he sure did. Since it was all on the house, I tasted every exotic dish possible with a gentle apology to my dad—surprising him in turn, but he understood.

We used to do a number of sorties from Hashi, spread over many days at a time, for BRO. Their headquarters for the Bhutan project were at Deothang. It was called Dantak. Quite often, we used to fly the chief engineer all the way to forward places like Tashi Gong Dzong. Sometimes, we got to fly the director-general of BRO, who used to come from Delhi. BRO did great work in pioneering road-building in the most inaccessible places in border areas opposite China. Today's extensive network of roads in Bhutan owes a lot to this effort.

Lodrai in the foothills was a refuelling point. It used to be done from barrels. This was a painstaking process to ensure quality control. Murphy's Law struck here in a most unusual way. A pilot in a Cheetah (light helicopter) had just positioned his chopper near the barrels and asked his co-pilot to start the switch-off procedure. He then realized that he had stopped on the wrong side and would run short of the fuel hose. So he raised power to laterally shift over the barrels to the other side. In the confusion, his co-pilot continued the switch-off drill—the result was that the chopper settled on the barrels! Fortunately, the crew re-engaged quickly, holding her gingerly on the barrels, thus salvaging the situation. In fact, they kept quiet about it. It only came to light a few weeks later, when the unit's CO was being complimented by a BRO senior officer on the skills of his pilots!

# UTTARI UTKRISHTI

TRANSLATED AS 'NORTHERN excellence', this chapter covers many states of northern and western India. But the focus is firmly on Jammu and Kashmir, including the militancy period in the Valley, and the saga of the Siachen Glacier, the highest battlefield in the world. No chopper pilot is complete unless he or she has operated in Ladakh. It is here that the biggest challenges lie for a military aviator.

Both man and machine gasp in the thin air while constantly being under threat of being shot down from the Pakistani side. The stories here cover the Kashmir valley from the time militancy raised its ugly head, the Kargil War, operations and adventures in Ladakh, and, of course, the Siachen Glacier. There are many untold and unsung stories of heroics and courage of the highest order, and life-defying-action tales that tested the limits of camaraderie. And all this under the most difficult conditions anywhere in the world.

## Vigil in the Valley

After Car Nicobar, I moved to Sarsawa, close to Saharanpur in Uttar Pradesh. It was my first tenure with the IAF's most versatile workhorse—the Mi-17 helicopter. Almost two years went by there with an overriding memory of operational detachments. It was the beginning of the 1990s and the IAF's helicopter fleet was in the thick of things such as the battle over Siachen and the burning insurgency in J&K, which had just assumed menacing proportions. My squadron, the Mighty Armours, had a finger in every pie. We had permanent detachments at Thoise, Ladakh, to support the Indian Army, and one at Srinagar in the armed role since none of our attack helicopters had crossed over Banihal Pass into the Kashmir valley till then. So it was quite the norm to come back after a month at one place, spend a day or two at home, which was for a long time a temporary two-room billet, and then be off for the next detachment. I am not even including numerous other assignments such as the Kullu Courier, a detachment at Kullu airport in Himachal Pradesh, to support governance when high mountain passes were closed due to snowfall.

### Versatile Vanguards

The Srinagar detachment was full of interesting stories with first-hand experience of the good and ugly side of managing J&K's uprising by the Indian government, and its trials and tribulations. It was but natural to be ready to support this effort in every conceivable way besides my primary role as an armed helicopter pilot. When fully armed with six rocket pods (192 rockets), a front gun and many other guns firing from side blisters, a Mi-17 is a truly potent weapon system. We used to go for firing practice to the nearby Toshe-Maidan range in the Shamshabad Mountains. As warriors, our fondest hope was to be employed in this role. And that day finally came in the spring of 1991. Passes had just opened and infiltration was going on as usual, despite the best efforts of the Indian Army. This was a time when the LoC had still not been fenced entirely. Army intelligence had homed in on a group of about fifty militants who had been trapped because of unusually heavy snowfall over the last two days. Since the army was finding it difficult to approach them, it was an ideal target for armed helicopters.

On getting our orders, we prepared for it. Airmen went to the aircraft in freezing temperatures before sunrise to laboriously load all 192 rockets and carry out other maintenance tasks. We too were there with our plans and maps ready, with all crew briefed and mock rehearsals done, ready to press the trigger. We finally took off by 10 a.m., delayed by the weather. However, fifteen minutes out, we were called back. On landing, our orders were to quickly reconfigure into a relief dropping mode. After a night's deliberations, and negotiations I suspect, Delhi and other powers that be had taken the decision of not taking out this group but helping them survive instead. So there we were, trigger-happy warriors, suitably chastened, dropping sleeping bags, blankets, food, ready-to-eat meals and other such life support items. We did not know whether to feel disappointed or elated. Like I said earlier, these were certainly trying times for the country and for us!

### A Silver Lining

A spin-off of the situation in the Valley was numerous invites to weddings and other social events from the high and mighty in Srinagar. That was not because of a sudden rise in our social status but security-related. Armed forces were welcomed, firstly because of a paucity of other guests afraid of being targeted, and then, security forces brought in inherent protection. I tasted my first 'wazwan' at the wedding of a very rich Kashmiri's daughter. I was not aware of the ritual of wazwan, and noticing the tiny morsel of meat in the first serving, I gestured for more. My friend sitting beside me, a NSG captain, told me to hang on for what was to follow. And follow it did—all thirty-six servings of meat dishes in the most savoury creations. I could barely clear my plate. Also, things became really cheap and affordable because of a virtual stop in tourism and business. Many items such as walnut wood furniture, badams or almonds, leather jackets and other lovely local products were available at dirt-cheap prices. Demands from the mainland multiplied. One could feel the desperation of the local community as normal life came to a near stop because of growing militancy. But their warm 'Kashmiriyat' was still very much alive.

## Back Again

After sixteen years, I was reposted to Badami Bagh, on the outskirts of Srinagar, as a TAC commander in the middle of the first decade of the new millennium. The situation was in relatively better control; however, action stations were still on with multiple encounters going on all across. The fence on the LoC had come up and the latest gizmos helped with better monitoring; however, the other side was equally tech-savvy and constantly innovating to surprise us. It was the first time the IAF's special force, or Garuds, were being exposed to combat along with the SF of the Indian Army. I used to coordinate many of these missions and, except for teething issues, they performed at par with their army comrades. We also tried out newer tactics of using Mi-17s and the SF to out-manoeuvre militant groups across the Shamshabad mountain ranges with a great degree of success.

Badami Bagh cantonment is the hub of the army's operations. It was fortified as nothing else could be. The threats were real and live every minute. Attempts to storm gates, scale walls and fidayeen attacks were common. I witnessed first-hand one such attempt. I was on the golf course with my army colleagues around 4 p.m. A distinct siren indicating a fidayeen attack was sounded. The entire station went into a lockdown drill that was perfect. Life came to a standstill in minutes and all guns were out. We simply jumped into a clump of bushes on the course to hide. Quick reaction teams neutralized the two infiltrators within half an hour. Another hour went in clearing and sanitizing the entire station, and then finally, the all-clear siren was sounded.

## The Other Foot

As I stated earlier, we were either in Srinagar or Siachen, if not involved in tougher locations. Siachen was a proper battle zone since the ceasefire had still not been declared. There was continuous shelling from both sides. Counterbattery, or taking out the enemy's artillery with your own, was a favourite tactic that resulted in constant shifting of base camps with all the attendant problems and nuisance value. Flying Mi-17s was as challenging as the real heroes—Siachen Pioneers in their Cheetahs. Most air maintenance drops had to be done with tactical manoeuvring to avoid getting into the direct line of fire of Pakistani guns. It almost meant that every getaway was a 'dicey' manoeuvre involving banking and engine power of the Mi-17 that the Russian manufacturer had not envisaged. Actually, we redefined the performance envelope of the helicopter from altitudes of just 4 km to 7 km above mean sea level—what better testing grounds! The danger was real—Nanda died when his Cheetah helicopter was shot, and Jain and his mates in a Mi-17 were fatally shot down. We used to warn other pilots of Pakistanis homing in on them by the expanding dark circles in the snow. These dark circles were shells or mortar that landed in deep snow and blossomed a while later.

Cheetah operations were even more demanding. I did these operations when flying with the Siachen Pioneers as part of the Aircrew Examining Board. Of course, I had more experience as the AOC in Leh later, when I flew both the Cheetah and Chital extensively in the glacier. But by that time, a ceasefire was on and combat risks were not as grave. You had to witness the antics that were indulged in many times a day. Who can think of a climbing approach to land and a backwards descending take-off from the highest helipad in the world! The size of landing sites are truly 'matchbox', and even a few inches here or there put you in grave vibrations or a chance to topple. You can't switch off, and only hand signals work in the noise to communicate with those on ground. An accident waiting to happen is an understatement; but nonetheless, chopper pilots have been doing this for more than three decades, professionally and safely.

## The Siachen Saga

Sometimes, peace is maintained at a heavy cost. Pakistani intrusions in the desolate high-altitude areas of Siachen in 1984 and the price India had to incur to counter this is a case in point. Such is the nature of the terrain that helicopters are the only lifeline for our gallant troops. The vast glaciated regions are perpetually snowbound and covered with mountains of ice. Strong winds, turbulence and extreme sub-zero temperature (minus 40 degrees Celsius) with white-outs hamper even routine operations. Helipads are at altitudes of 4.5 to 5.2 km above mean sea level, which makes helicopter operations difficult and dangerous with very little reserves of power. More often than not, pilots fly hugging the few valleys and barely clear the ridges that are usually covered with clouds. The world's highest battlefield, sustained for many decades, is truly a tribute to IAF helicopter crews.

Operation Meghdoot was launched on 13 April 1984. It was planned in support of the Indian Army and paramilitary forces in northern Ladakh to secure control of the heights dominating the Siachen Glacier; also referred to as the world's third pole and potentially a dangerous flashpoint on the disputed northern borders. The Indian Army permanently stationed over 2,000 men all along the 110-km-long Actual Ground Position Line (AGPL). Over decades, the IAF's transport fleet of IL-76s, An-12s and An-32s transported stores and troops, and airdropped supplies to high altitudes; while helicopters like Mi-17s, Mi-8s, Chetaks and Cheetahs ferried men and material to dizzying heights, far above the limits set by helicopter manufacturers. In fighting for this 'roof of the world' since then, an incredible aviation performance in extreme temperature and altitude has become a benchmark for the world. A most inhospitable region, it contains some of the highest peaks. It is the second-longest glacier outside the polar region with a length of 76 km. The area is mountainous, rugged, precipitous and glacial with heights varying from 12,000 to 24,000 feet. It remains snowbound with sub-zero temperatures throughout the year. Poor visibility creates problems of navigation, coupled with high-velocity winds, especially after mid-day. The whole concoction makes flying an extremely hazardous and difficult task.

## Believe It or Not

I once landed in Puh, a forward helipad in Himachal Pradesh. We had about two hours to kill on ground and I got chatting with an army coursemate who was posted there. He told us of a chopper—a Mi-17 landing on a road stretch that was impossible to be replicated ever. I challenged that, knowing well that my flight commander Deshu had done a precautionary landing a few weeks back, but reported it as nothing unusual. Curiosity and an argument with my coursemate finally made us drive to the place just 20 km away. It was unbelievably small with a rock face on one side and a sheer drop on the other. The army unit had embedded a plaque that stated: 'Believe it or not—a Mi-17 helicopter landed here.' They had marked the spots where the three wheels had touched. The one near the sheer drop was just six inches away. The rotor blade near the rock face had been inches away. In fact, before starting the next morning, soldiers had to manually chip off a foot deep of the rock face for safety—it took six hours to do this. It meant that the landing had been '*bhagwan bharose*', or literally in the hands of God! Deshu and Delta had to do this because they got caught in a blizzard trying to reach Puh.

## The Fastest CASEVAC

The parachute drop area near Sarsawa was a familiar spot with both the air force adventure team and the official para school guys coming at regular intervals to practise from our Mi-17s. One Sunday, I was captaining a sortie with the para school team practising. A Groupie, Rath, from Air HQ, who was once a member of the para school, was also going along for his revalidation. As the final stick of para-jumpers exited, my gunner from the cargo compartment called out that a parachutist was in trouble. A rare collapse of one side of the chute due to tangling had taken place, and the jumper was spiralling down. One of the team members on board reported it as critical. I descended, keeping a little away from the track of all the jumpers. We spotted the chute and the immobile figure away from the dropping zone. We landed next to it and everybody available, except me on controls, went to assist. The motionless jumper was gingerly put on a stretcher and into the helicopter. We took off and radioed Sarsawa to inform Delhi that we were getting a serious case to the Base Hospital (BH) there. Reaching there in forty minutes, it was gratifying to see the ambulance waiting at the helipad close to the BH. It was probably the fastest helicopter casualty pick-up ever—it saved Rath's life.

## Safed Sagar

In 1999, our traditional adversary, Pakistan, carried out a misadventure on a mammoth scale in the Kargil–Dras sector. Regular Pakistani army troops came and occupied many peaks and ridges overlooking Kargil and Dras in the guise of militants. It went largely unnoticed until the occupation reached its critical threshold. Pakistani forces were now present in positions of advantage, overlooking most of the national highway 1-A, and directly threatening the Kargil valley. The Indian Army swung into action and carried out several assaults, incurring heavy casualties due to the tactical disadvantage of having to carry out operations in continuous view of the adversary positioned above. It was soon realized that air operations were imperative to flush out these intruders. The IAF pooled in all resources and initiated Operation Safed Sagar. In the initial days of the operation, a Mi-17 helicopter was lost to enemy fire. Flt Lt Muhilan, one of the helicopter martyrs who had been a Siachen Tiger, gave the supreme sacrifice and laid down his life in the icy heights of Dras sector.

With tensions increasing, the rest of us were on standby to move to the northern sector. Everyone was more than keen to move into operations. Air maintenance was stopped and helicopters were fitted with rocket pods. Two pilots from the Siachen Tigers, which I was commanding, were attached to Sarsawa to take part—Ahlu and Verma had moved to Srinagar and were flying extensively in the entire area spanning from Srinagar to Leh. Sorties were primarily aimed at casualty evacuation and army mobilization. In addition, a massive air effort was put in to deliver supplies, including ammunition, to soldiers deployed on the war front. On 9 June, information was received that four more Tigers had to go to Srinagar, which was followed by a rush to the flight commander's office with all aircrew volunteering for the task. Finally, on 11 June, the four lucky pilots—Robin, Kathuria, Manish and Dobhal—were launched to Guwahati from where they were airlifted to Srinagar to fly in Operation Safed Sagar. I joined them a week later. We operated from the golf course at Badami Bagh in the heart of Srinagar, and flew many missions braving enemy fire and going up to the far reaches in the theatre of operations. As many as 220 battle casualties were evacuated, some under extremely hostile conditions. The airlift of four extremely heavy 105 mm artillery guns to Chakwali in Gurez sector, in a single day and under enemy shelling, was a feather in our cap—the story comes a little later. We did numerous missions with the SF, including to Bakarwal and Kaobal Gali under enemy fire. In fact, the para-commando operations depicted in the movie *Lakshya* actually involved 6 Para and us. Of course, considerable artistic licence has been resorted to in the movie—the reality was quite different.

## Casualty Evacuation: Kargil 1999

I am going to now share some actual wartime experiences of handling battle casualties. It is also a reality check for tech-savvy youngsters who believe that technology is the answer to all problems. Battle casualties, and I mean the injured or maimed and not the dead, are a grave tactical reality. It is planned by adversaries, especially in the mountains, because of a simple fact—an injured soldier requires the dedicated effort of four people over many days for evacuation. This takes away vital manpower, which is anyway a criticality in the mountains. Evacuation is, in turn, important for morale. Otherwise, soldiers will not venture forward. It was key to the heroics performed by Indian soldiers, especially in Kargil.

The first story took place at Zoji La Pass, or Gumri, which was the site of a field ambulance hospital housed in tents. It served as the main base for triage and life support for critical cases before they could be air-evacuated to the Srinagar military hospital. Incidentally, the road from Srinagar to Zoji La was completely blocked by trucks, all standing bumper-to-bumper, to supply the Indian Army's requirements. Air evacuation was the only way out. I was the CO of a squadron that evacuated nearly 220 casualties from Gumri. Most of these were because of air bursts from artillery shells, from which there was no protection on a steep mountain slope. I was surprised to see so many critical cases. However, surprise turned to shock when I found out that only one surgeon was available throughout the war at that place.

I met him while he was at surgery. He was half-asleep! He claimed to be on his feet almost twenty hours every day. It was unbelievable that more surgeons could not be spared at Gumri. The next shock was the scarcity of stretchers. The CO of the field ambulance unit refused to let go of the stretchers for fear of accounting. I promised that we would return them on the next trip. In fact, we had an ugly argument on the issue, but he did not relent. The attendants would get a patient to the Mi-17 and just roll him on to the floor (covered in blankets) by tilting the stretcher. They were doing this by the hundreds! Drip bottles and other such fixtures were just tied up to any support available within the helicopter. The sheer numbers and pressure of time did not allow any improvements.

The second story was in the Gurez Valley, the western-most point in the Kargil War. The army wanted to put pressure from the flanks by capturing a Pakistani post called Laila-Majnu Tila. In the first attempt around 4 a.m., it suffered huge casualties. All the manpower was used up in bringing back the dead and injured, and it took two days to do this. The next day, in consultation with the brigade commander, I engaged my two Mi-17s in an unbelievable saga of forty-seven short hops to drop four 105 mm artillery guns (dismantled) at the high-altitude helipad of Chakwali. Actually, there was no helipad, only a dried-up stream in the narrowest of valleys imaginable. Many of these sorties were out of the limits of the performance of my helicopter. But war is war and improvisation is the answer. It was almost sunset by the time I finished the last sortie. The guns had been put together and had already started firing at Pakistani bunkers (or sangars). That night, the battalion (Gurkhas) walked over the post with no casualties, since the guns had destroyed all enemy bunkers.

But the real story is what happened after I landed at Chakwali with the last gun part. I had enough fuel to go back to Srinagar. A captain approached me with a request to take three critical casualties and one body being brought down from the first attack two days ago. I was running out of time and fuel, since the engines were running. After five minutes, I called the officer and expressed my inability to wait any more. As I opened throttle, the battalion's subedar major stood in front of the helicopter with his hands folded and head bowed, begging me to wait. What really stopped me was a Gurkha soldier beside him, his rifle pointing at me! The captain came in and apologetically said that the situation was out of his control. We finally waited for twenty minutes and the only thing that stopped me from switching off there and then was the altitude, at which a Mi-17 could never be restarted. As I was taking off, the guns paused so that we could pass through safely. Night flying in mountainous valleys was prohibited, but I had no choice. In the confusing shadows and darkness, I crossed the Razdan Pass at a height of over 15,000 feet with a silent prayer on my lips. This was without any oxygen, and I rate it as one of my most demanding and risk-fraught missions. Srinagar had raised an overdue alert thinking we had crashed! We landed at Badami Bagh helipad by night, from where the critical cases were immediately shifted for surgery and all were saved. I got a warning from the authorities at Srinagar for the whole episode, but thankfully I was not grounded. All in all, emotions run high during war. I never reported the indiscretions of the Gurkhas.

### War Vignettes

As the Kargil War started, there was great outpouring of support for the armed forces from across the country. But there was great pressure too on the army's leadership for allowing such a surprise to crop up in the first place. Rightfully, it got into overdrive to address the anomaly. During one visit of the army chief, he couldn't help but notice some officers playing golf in the afternoon at the Badami Bagh course. This may have been because of an earlier damning media report on the issue. The orders were immediate and clear—no more golf. The fallout was that six Mi-17s were told to move and operate from the Badami Bagh Cantonment golf course. We used to land on the gentle greens, especially the flat ones—they were firmer than the long fairways with trees lined up. Imagine the damage we did. Later in life when I took to golf, I regretted it and had nightmares about the damage done to such a beautiful course.

An army moves on its stomach—how true! From our choppers we could see hundreds of trucks, full of supplies, stuck on the national highway right up to Zoji La. In fact, many of them reached only after the war. An unintended but tasty fallout was that some of the goodies sent by benefactors fell on us to consume. A businessman from Saharanpur had sent two trucks laden with crates of ripe mangoes for the front. These had to be distributed in Srinagar itself since they would never find their way to the border. The next two days were spent eating only mangoes, with the choicest varieties from Uttar Pradesh. Unfortunately, it had a telling effect on our tummies. Thankfully, we had enough spare aircrew.

## Ladakh Disaster 2010

In August 2010, the entire mountain range around Leh received unusually high rainfall. This area, normally referred to as a desert, has mountains that are not made to withstand excessive water flow, a key constituent being mud and rocks that come apart if wet. Wise locals lament government efforts of greening pockets such as Leh, Nimu, and others. Many locals claim that even the Dalai Lama has said that greenery attracts clouds, and that rains are an ecological disaster. What Ladakhis want is good snowfall, which ensures a slow but perennial supply of water in the small streams and canals that feed the land and its people.

Anyway, what was inevitable happened on 6 August. All over Ladakh, large mudslides virtually took out huge chunks of mountain slopes and cascaded into the Indus. All bridges and roads to Leh were cut off. Leh town was badly affected with half of it wiped out. That included the large and only civil hospital, the BSNL communications centre that was the node for telecommunications, the only runway and the adjoining suburb of Choglamsar. With no mobile and telephone connectivity, no flights and no vehicular movement, Leh became a ghost town. It was still tourist season with hundreds of trekking parties stuck all over. Many people had been killed, but more importantly, there were many injured who required evacuation and medical aid. Delhi was clueless as to how to get aid into Leh. I was deputed as the task force commander from the IAF to attend the crisis management multi-agency meetings in South Block.

The first requirement was situational awareness and getting the Leh airbase back on its feet. The IAF and Indian Army joined hands to clear the runway manually. At the same time, rescue and medical aid efforts were on in full swing at Leh by all agencies. Within thirty-six hours, the first IL-76 started to land on a just about acceptable runway. Six more followed quickly with teams and equipment to speed up the rescue phase. The first two days were spent on receiving military and civil flights bringing in supplies and taking out those stranded. However, our foreign ministry in Delhi was getting hundreds of calls from embassies demanding help for trekkers who were stuck. Some had got in touch with their countries through satellite phones. The problem was that exact locations were not known.

The importance of multi-agency meetings at Delhi became quite evident on the third day of the effort. BSNL officers had been calling for carriage of heavy equipment to revive telecommunications at Leh. But no one listened since priorities were different. The J&K government's resident commissioner had clearly drawn the priority for tents and other associated equipment to rehabilitate townspeople in light of the approaching winter. Embassies were still clamouring for rescuing trekking teams. In all the heated debates, I simply pointed out that reviving telecommunications was the only way we could have a coherent rescue and rehabilitation effort. The group allowed me to prioritize—and we did with the next five IL-76 sorties of BSNL heavy equipment from Chandigarh. Within twenty-four hours, the BSNL network came up, initially on a temporary basis. Suddenly, all teams could be tracked and helicopter evacuations started in right earnest with both the IAF and army choppers at full throttle.

One incident stands out. Our foreign ministry was pushing for the evacuation of foreign nationals. One could understand the stakes involved in terms of credibility, reputation and international relationships. A group of ninety-six trekkers had converged in a valley, at the confluence of two torrential streams. Emergency rations had been dropped earlier. Now the pressure was to evacuate them from that difficult spot where a small chopper could get in but not land. A joint secretary very uncharacteristically barked out the demand of evacuating the ninety foreigners, invoking the highest level of the government. When I queried about the six local porters, his reply was, 'Not my business, just take out the ninety foreigners.' I was seething with rage but held back to do what I had to do. I got in touch with Patel, the CO of the Siachen Pioneers in Leh. We planned out the sorties with six Cheetah light helicopters. In the first wave, some helpers were to be dropped to control the non-stop effort to follow. However, my final directions were to pick up the six Indian porters in the first wave. And that is exactly how it happened. Only two persons could be picked up in one chopper, and therefore many sorties were done by the six helicopters. By evening the job was done, beamed real-time on TV across the world. I made sure the government official got to know what I had done, but he never got back. All embassies involved wrote to the Chief of Air Staff (CAS) in glowing terms of the IAF's commitment and professionalism.

Rehabilitation and support to the locals continued throughout the winter. A temporary township based on winter tents saw the locals through the harsh winter. When I went to Leh as AOC two years later, the first thing I did was to uproot hundreds of saplings that had been planted in the base as a 'greening' drive—once bitten, twice shy. The top man of BSNL on a visit to Leh called in at my office. He seemed to be aware of what had happened in 2010 and presented me a small plaque with a very interesting quote written on it: 'I do not believe in a fate that falls on men however they act; but I do believe in a fate that falls on them unless they act.'

## Camaraderie Redefined

I have written somewhere else about my close association with General Bakshi, who was the corps commander in 2012–13. It ran deep based on mutual trust and faith in each other's intent. There were many instances when this came to the fore, especially during the stand-offs with the Chinese army in Ladakh. There were also many cases where my pilots put their own lives on the line to save soldiers—and the army reciprocated. No better examples to illustrate this than the two true tales that follow.

Khardung La Pass is rated as not only the highest motorable pass in the world but also the most difficult to manoeuvre, especially in winters. Night-driving during snowfall around the pass is prohibited for the military. Two of my airmen were coming back from the Siachen Glacier and decided to hitch a ride in a taxi since the military convoy had gone and the next one was only on the following day. All was okay till the beginning of the climb at Khalsar. Heavy snowfall was reported and the prudent thing for the Ladakhi driver would have been to call things off, but he persisted. An even more prudent thing for my airmen would have been to give up on the non-refundable fare and catch a convoy the next day. But because one of them had his leave and a seat in the courier (IL-76), they decided to quietly go against the orders prohibiting night movement. They started having trouble midway at North Pullu, encountering difficult snowy conditions. All plans went awry, and night descended. Now it was a do-or-die mode since stopping at above 15,000 feet would have killed them anyway with temperature dipping way below zero degrees. They persisted, sliding from side to side in just the vehicle's headlights. It was almost 10 p.m. when suddenly the Ladakhi driver lost control and the vehicle plunged down from nearly 17,000 feet. Just before that, the driver jumped out and saved himself. The vehicle hurtled down to sure doom; however, heavy snow stopped the fall 1,000 feet down. The taxi had crumpled, trapping both the airmen. One had fractured his leg and was caught under some metal distortion. They risked freezing to death trapped at 15,000 feet, or one of them could have bled to death. The driver would get back after many hours but, being a Ladakhi, his genes allowed him to survive the night ordeal. The last skewer was that the area was in a blind zone with no mobile network. So no one could know what had happened.

In Ladakh, one gets a feeling of being closer to God, both figuratively and physically. The two airmen, without any hope and in desperation, gave a blind call on their mobiles to a colleague back at the Leh base. After a few tries, miraculously and by some freak atmospheric phenomenon, he got through with just enough time to explain his predicament. Thereafter, despite hundreds of attempts, there was 'no joy'.

By the time I was woken up, it was already approaching midnight. After taking stock, I decided to call General Bakshi, despite the army exchange saying he couldn't be disturbed and never had been in his tenure. I finally got through and all the great man said was, 'Rajesh, don't worry. I have the controls.' A great rescue past midnight was launched, which involved a team rappelling (if that can be done on snow) down 1,000 feet, carrying metal-cutting equipment, first aid, special thermal stretchers, and so on. Finally, around 3 a.m., the boys were pulled up to the special ambulance, given emergency resuscitation and taken to North Pullu. They were kept under intensive care till early morning, when we moved them in a chopper to Partapur Hospital for proper care. They did survive to talk about the miracle. I was overwhelmed but got a gentle rebuke when I started thanking the general profusely, who simply said that we all had done our duty.

The story does not end there. A few months later, an army ALH (light helicopter) took off from Leh for Siachen Glacier.

After a regular sortie, it faced technical problems coupled with bad weather. Somehow the pilots managed to crash-land on the main glacier. It was critical to rescue them from exposure since ground parties would take at least twenty-four hours to traverse multiple crevasses and mountains of ice blocks. It would be too late. Now the general rang up and I repeated his own words to him about controls with me. I spoke to my pilot at the base camp, Harvey, who said this could be done only as a single-pilot configuration. I cleared him and told him to do it from the nearest helipad (Qazi). But I did express reservations about how the surviving pilots, sapped of energy and oxygen, would climb to a hovering Chital in its downwash. He came back after much calculations and deliberation that a two-pilot configuration was just okay, with the other helping the survivors to come in. The go-ahead was given for the mission. In two very careful and risky shuttles, both downed pilots were rescued and transported to intensive care. They too survived to tell a great tale. I was finally even with Rajan Bakshi—my good friend! After all, a friend in need is a friend indeed. Harvey was awarded a Shaurya Chakra for his gallant act.

### Baba Mehar

Here is a legend that Indians can be proud of. Baba Mehar's exploits as a fighter pilot got him the highest awards of the country, but it was his service in J&K in 1947–48, flying Dakotas, that the country is truly indebted to. The landing at a 600-yard ALG at Poonch, and the timely delivery of troops of the Indian Army at Srinagar are legendary stuff. A similar effort was done by the first-ever landing at Leh on 24 May 1948. Pakistani infiltrators had reached Nimu, just 30 km away from Leh. The reinforcements brought in by Baba and his gang in hundreds of sorties finally pushed them away beyond Kargil—Leh was saved and history was made.

The airbase at Leh has a bust of Baba Mehar overlooking the main dispersal from where Leh has been air-maintained for the last seven decades. Diametrically opposite the dispersal, in the Zanskar mountain range, is a pyramid-shaped peak. It towers over the airbase as if protecting it under its wings. I decided to launch a climbing expedition to scale this in February 2014. It was flagged off by Air Chief Marshal Arup Raha. After scaling it in an arduous three-day climb over rock and snow, we did a puja and christened it 'Baba Mehar Peak'.

There is a small hill right next to the runway that houses the Spituk Monastery at the top. It is of great importance to Ladakhi culture and has a history of being visited by greats such as Nehru, Indira Gandhi and many others. I developed a special relationship with the head monk and other priests there. We offered help in many ways. An annual feature was the monastery festival in the thick of winters, the only monastery to do so in a non-tourist season. Since it was one of a kind, it was very popular all over Ladakh. But all roads and passes were closed so supplies to support this two-day effort were just not feasible, especially fresh vegetables. As a special gesture, we used to fly them in as part of our supplies and provide them as an offering. I would not only be invited as an esteemed guest; but the monastery would also say special prayers for the airbase.

## Unique Ladakh

A similar strong affiliation was built with the Ladakh Scouts Regimental Centre (LSRC)—a regiment that boasts more than 300 gallantry awards. These were men who were built for high-altitude work and who needed no acclimatization. For mainlanders like us, a three-stage process spread over almost ten days is required to stay and operate above 15,000 feet. Their logo was a wild mountain goat, the ibex, and they were as sure-footed on mountain slopes as these animals. While we gave them special privileges at the airbase, they provided us help all across Ladakh during various operational deployments and adventure expeditions. I was a special guest during their golden jubilee Raising Day, where I ensured that about 50 kg of fresh laddus from Chandigarh flew in on time for the scouts and their families.

Many of our airmen were deployed on the glacier at the highest posts. To make them feel special, and as a motivation to volunteer for such tasks, the maximum commendations and awards were reserved for them. When back at the airbase, they were made to retain their beards for a couple of days to allow public recognition. Any opportunity to felicitate such youngsters was never missed out. Importantly, their stories allowed empathy to grow for all those serving up there. It was amusing to see air force personnel giving preferences in couriers or seats in other aircraft to the 'glacier-returned'. Public announcements were made to identify such jawans.

Snow clearances were great community activities. Leh runway being the only lifeline in winters, everyone was more than happy to help. Despite many state-of-the-art snow removers, at least 500 people used to descend following a well-laid-out procedure to clear the snow for incoming IL-Babas. Surprisingly, there are only about four to five spells of heavy snowfall in the valley. Up in the mountains and the passes, it snowed almost every day during winters.

Air Chief Marshal Raha made his first visit to Leh after taking over as CAS in January 2014. It was the thick of winter and temperatures plummeted to minus 20 degrees or less. He came in special extreme-cold clothing and decided that the cocktails with the army also should be in fatigues—it was too cold to change. The next morning, before returning to Delhi, he addressed all personnel of the base in a hangar that was not heated. The temperature was minus 17 degrees as he stood on the rostrum, and standing behind him, I could make out how uncomfortable he was. But overall, it was a great morale booster for the airmen that the CAS's first visit was to their station.

Elections in Ladakh are truly different from those held anywhere else in the country. In 2014, Discovery Channel covered the marvel of Indian elections in a full documentary. A sizeable part was the coverage in the difficult, remote and inaccessible parts of Ladakh, which can only be covered by a sizeable number of small helicopters. We used to start preparations a few months earlier so that the maximum numbers of choppers with sufficient flying hours were available in that short period of three days. The spoiler was weather, of course, but if it held, sorties were carried out at breakneck speed and throughout the day. There was a village that required two choppers to fly for two hours to reach it, with just ten voters. But our great Election Commission was clear—everyone had to have a chance to exercise his or her franchise.

The Dalai Lama does not visit Leh too often. He came for the Kal Chakra, a major prayer meeting spread over a month in 2014. But just before that, he came to Leh to visit Padam on the Zanskar River. When he came to board his helicopter, I was there as AOC to see him off. I had flown him way back in 1999 to Tawang. He looked much older, but his eyes were as bright as ever. His spiritual aura is indescribable and bathes everything around him in calmness and serenity. Of course, he had not lost his wonderful sense of humour. He clasped my hand around the thumb and held on till he boarded his helicopter—a full twenty minutes. After he had gone, all the high and mighty figures of Ladakh politics and administration present wanted to touch my hand that His Holiness had clasped. They insisted that I had been blessed! When he returned from Padam, after seeking permission, we allowed some family members of the base to meet him and take selfies.

The first Leh marathon was to be organized in September 2012. It was a big international event recognized by appropriate world sports bodies. The organizers along with members of the local administration came to meet me for some help. One of the mandatory requirements in the mountains is the availability of chopper evacuation plans, but there were no civilian ones around to be employed. Also, it would be prohibitively expensive, with no time left to sign a contract. I advised the district commissioner that since he was empowered to solicit casualty evacuation for all of Ladakh from the IAF on a payment basis, he could use that as an evacuation cover. He did so and the administration was overjoyed.

The event took place and was a grand success. In the series of runs, the Khardung La Challenge is unique among marathons. It starts from Khardung village, north of the famed pass, before sunrise. Crossing over the pass, a total of 72 km has to be covered. A Ladakh Scout jawan won the first two marathons that I remember. I was invited to do the 10 km run towards the pass and back. I did and clocked fifty-eight minutes, which was a very good timing. A special medal for my timing, and for being the oldest participant, was a delightful end at the large public function. I did notice that thereafter the local administration was very responsive to IAF land acquisition processes.

The eighteen-hole golf course at Leh is truly one of a kind. The clubhouse is perched at about 11,000 feet and the highest tee-off is at 13,000 feet above mean sea level. Even acclimatized golfers run out of breath climbing up and are forced to take a short break. And only then the fabulous panoramic view of Leh, nestled in the mountains with Khardung La in the backdrop, hits you. It takes your breath away! There are no greens—only sand mixed with oil 'browns'. But the truly memorable experience was playing in the winters with Leh painted white with snow. Despite bright-coloured balls, it was difficult to find your ball. The trick was to look for its entry point—a clear neat hole in the snow—and dig it out from there.

## Circle of Zanskar

In September 1987, I had come for a rafting expedition to Leh from Jaisalmer in Rajasthan. Our guide was Yusuf Zaheer, a schoolmate and the son of late Air Marshal Jafar Zaheer. We did some practice runs on the Indus for a week and then started for Padam via Kargil in a military truck. It was an arduous journey till Kargil, where we spent the night and bought some provisions. The next day was a risky drive to Rangdum Monastery where we spent the night. It was an early start the next morning since we had to clear Pensi La Pass before 2 p.m. In the entire stretch, till our halting point beyond the pass, we did not cross any other vehicle. It was that desolate and lonely. But the scenic beauty was absolutely out of this world. Bushes full of orange-coloured Leh berries gave way to rhododendrons and finally no flora at all. At Pensi La, the snout of the glacier could be explored—it was so close to the road. After a cold night halt, we reached Padam in the late afternoon, crossing and driving along many streams and rivers, including the torrential Suru river.

There were just five of us and a sixteen-foot raft. We gave ourselves a rest day to explore Padam and its famed monastery up on a remote hill. The next day, we set course on the Zanskar and its famed gorges. It took us six days to reach Nimu with five night camps in complete wilderness. The gorges are awe-inspiring vertical walls rising to 20,000 feet from the valley bottom, itself at 14,000 feet. It can make one dizzy just looking up. At one point, the river narrowed to just 20 feet—it was scary. Later on, I would come to learn that this was the site of Neraq village, which was cut off from the rest of the world for most parts of the year except winters. That was the time the river froze on top and allowed villagers to commute to Leh on the 'Chadar', as it is then called.

While most rapids were between grades three and four, we came across one that was a sure five. We stopped and anchored to study and plan our traversing. Sheer vertical walls on either side ensured that we used our rock-climbing skills to reach near the rapids. We were completely crestfallen—it looked impossible even after studying it for two hours. The dilemma was that neither could we portage, meaning carry the raft via the bank across, nor could we go back. Finally, Zaheer made a plan and we went for it. I have been a sportsman all my life and am no stranger to the flow of adrenalin. But I distinctly remember the overflow of adrenalin—heart in my mouth and every other sensation that comes when grave danger is ahead.

Initially, all went as per plan. However, as we came across the main section, all hell broke loose. The oars were snatched from Zaheer's hands and he dived forward saying, 'Guys, remember high side.' It meant put weight on to whichever side was coming up to stop high waves from flipping us over. We stretched half out of the raft and put all our weight on that side. Somehow we made it out, totally out of control! It was so sapping that we went for the nearest campsite just half a kilometre away to get back to normal. At the campfire that night, hardly anyone spoke.

On the final run, as we were nearing the confluence, we noticed quite a crowd, shamianas (colourful tents) and vehicles. Suddenly, two IAF officers in uniform (khaki in those days) rushed to us. One was the AOC himself. They were yelling at us, asking how we came in so early (11 a.m.). We were quite perplexed and I went out to meet him. The story was that the vice-chief from Delhi was coming to flag us in. Without a clue about what we had done, he explained that it was the talk of the town in Delhi—the pioneering rafting expedition on the Zanskar. Then he asked us to go back and come only when we got a signal. How do you go back in a raft against a powerful river? But the AOC would not relent and maintained that we were spoiling the show.

We finally pulled the raft 200 metres upstream to hide behind a large rock face on the Indus. We did get our promised tea and biscuits, secretly of course.

Around 2 p.m., we got the signal and rafted in to a befitting climax. Many photographs and speeches later, we finally managed to attack a sumptuous meal with the vice-chief. He did compliment us on our feat, as also our appetites. Back in Delhi, more shock awaited us. Zaheer was given a warning by an international rafting association that carried weight for going on such a dangerous mission without accompanying rafts and kayaks for rescue. It seemed that an American expedition of two rafts had attempted the same two years ago. One raft and its occupants never survived and were never found. The entire expedition had wound up halfway. Had we known this, I would never have conceived of it, let alone attempt it! Now, let me fast forward to a full quarter of a century later.

As an AOC, I dreamt of doing a Chadar trek up the frozen River Zanskar. After meticulous preparation, the team was ready, led by a lady officer, Rachika, an Everester from the famous IAF all-women expedition. We prepared our sleds that are pulled along with shoulder straps (aka rucksacks) on top. This is done to avoid dangerous broken ice on the river when one has to pick up and haul them over one's shoulders to manoeuvre the rock faces. We had taken two doctors and medicines to organize health camps at villages along the route. The plan was to trek up to Padam and come back to Nimu. A number of tourist teams also undertake the well-organized tour but only for two days. Ours was an eleven-day expedition. Temperatures plummet to minus 30 degrees with winds sometimes reaching blizzard strength in the night. The whole experience was great—almost surreal, and I recommend it to all those with adventure in their blood.

## A Bridge Too Far!

I must now focus on Neraq, a village that is almost midway between Leh and Padam. As I described in my rafting story earlier, it used to be cut off for most parts of the year. There are no children in the village since all of them are at boarding schools in Leh and only come back for winter holidays (a full two months) via the Chadar. At the narrowest gorge section, there was a wooden bridge made of logs, without any railing. The villagers had put it up themselves to be used only in an emergency. I spent a full day and night with the villagers, staying with my chief host who had met and invited me in Leh. Local cultural events and a very potent brew followed, and there was great merry-making. The next morning, before I left and since they sought nothing in return, I asked the village elders if there was anything that I could do. They requested me to pressure the administration at Leh to build a proper iron bridge for the people.

Once back, I met the district commissioner (DC), Simrandeep, a very positive man. He was a good friend and, being from the Rashtriya Indian Military College, had great empathy for the services. The problem was not only funds and procurement but how to get most of the stuff across to the Neraq side. Everyone pitched in—the army with some funds and bridge equipment, NGOs, private parties with additional funds, some equipment was brought in by IAF aircraft. After almost six months, it was all ready and stored at Nimu. From there it was under-slung and put first across the bridge foundation. Much of the stuff was dropped at the helipad from where villagers pitched in to shoulder it to the river side. Almost a year after my stay at Neraq, the bridge was complete and inaugurated. The DC and I were real heroes to the people of Neraq; however, the joy was short-lived.

As fate would have it, on 31 December 2014, an artificial blockage got created upstream of Padam, at Phutkal. As the ensuing 5 km artificial lake enlarged, worries of devastation downstream in case it broke increased. Finally, an informed decision was taken to blast it in phases, in a controlled manner. People were moved to safer heights on the due dates in May 2015. It was an overall success; however, the Neraq bridge, hardly a year old, was washed away. Neraq villagers were promised a new one, but I was sceptical about anyone having the passion to see it through like Simrandeep. I was wrong—a new bridge did come up in late 2017.

### Tashi's Neraq

Our Chadar trek was made more memorable by a chance meeting with Tashi. He was from Neraq but worked in Leh as a part of the administration. He had a traditional house built in true Ladakhi style that I spent two days in at Neraq. The village is at an elevation of 15,000 feet above sea level. The snow was almost up to our knees, even after clearance, and yet the zest for life and traditions was palpable in everyone. Tashi's family witnessed the bridge-building efforts over the years. I was not only accepted as an honorary member of the village elders' group; my framed photo finds a pride of place in the community hall—it definitely is a singular honour.

Besides the bridging effort and annual medical camp by the IAF, we started numerous other initiatives to help the villagers of Zanskar. A boarding school that primarily catered to them at Leh was supported by us. I also organized fun-filled trips for children to the airbase. Many of the girls especially vowed to join the IAF. I coerced my good friend, Shri Spalbar, the chairman of Ladakh Autonomous Hill Development Council, to release additional scholarships for the Zanskaris. Plenty of IAF souvenir goodies were much-sought-after items among the children.

It was with Tashi that I first saw a snow leopard in the mountains. He spotted it easily, but I took time to home in on it. It was my only sighting of this rare animal and I truly cherish it.

The villagers of Neraq still keep in touch with me through Tashi's mobile and WhatsApp. The women of Neraq knitted a woollen robe for me with their own hands. It is maroon in colour—the same that monks and village elders wear.

## Legendary Loadmasters

The IL-76, or IL-Baba, has done yeoman service for almost three decades. Just like its predecessors the An-12, Packet (with an additional engine retrofitted on top) and the Dakota. Among all these, the IL-76 came in as a game changer because of its power and carrying capacity. Yet, in the 'hot and high' times of summer, even an IL-76 finds it difficult to carry anything back, sometimes actually nothing! This, despite the fact that Leh has one of the longest runways in India—a full 12,000 feet.

The arrival of the C-130J Super Hercules saw another change in the game. While it does not carry as much as a fully loaded IL-76, it retains its usual capacity through the entire temperature range at Leh. It also demonstrated its full capacity at Kargil where only An-32s could land with load limitations. But the icing on the cake was the demonstration of operations at Daulat Beg Oldie (DBO). Before that, my team at Leh and DBO were busy for almost two months, levelling and preparing the kutcha runway. I did repeated trips in helicopters to inspect the work and also spent an out-of-the-world three days at DBO. This required an acclimatization routine of seven days since I was already first-stage acclimatized.

Before all this could sink in, another game changer arrived—the C-17 heavy lifter. It redefined everything about operations at Leh. However, it couldn't leave the main runway since its outboard engines could pick up sand and get damaged. No problem, though—what was supposed to be a multi-crore solution of extending the paved areas was made into a simple one costing only a few lakhs. After preparation of the ground, river stones—round ones of similar sizes abundant in the Indus—were laid out neatly, and then cement slurry was poured on it, all levelled out. This allowed manual cleaning but no vehicles on it. The smart and temporary solution has lasted hundreds of C-17 sorties regularly for years. We were also on a fast learning curve to turn around the C-17 for its return with passengers. From the initial six hours, we finally nailed it down to a forty-five-minute standard procedure. Jointness between the army and air force was at its best. Did I mention that a unique feature of Leh runway is a 1,000-foot elevation difference between the two ends? Such are operations at the roof of the world.

As one lands in Leh, a towering mountainside with a sand-filled hollow catches one's attention because of a clear bold message written across: 'Touch the sky with glory.' This is right over a large IAF emblem. It is all pierced together with perforated steel sheets that once made the runway surface. Over decades, the runway graduated to a firm concrete-cum-road finish; however, some remnants of the old runway are still kept as an everlasting legacy. These sheets were laboriously taken on to the mountain to be fixed in the sand as a message. They were then painted white to always stand out. All this was done by personnel of the station itself. Every year, just before Air Force Day on 8 October, a large complement of picnickers, including visiting families, trudge up the mountain of knee-deep sand to touch up the sheets with paint. It is a beautiful moment dedicated to the IAF's great legacy of saving and sustaining Ladakh.

# ADBHUT ANDAMAN AND NICOBAR

THIS IS A short section that captures the unique backdrop of India's farthest island chain, one of our most strategic possessions. Readers will get a taste of the tribal cultures of the Holchus, the Sentinelese (alleged to be hostile and cannibalistic), the Onges (pygmies) and the peaceful Shompens, covering the entire chain as seen from a pilot's eyes.

There are stories of rescue at sea from a drifting ship amidst towering monsoon waves, and also some snippets of the post-tsunami rescue and relief. There are also some tales involving the supernatural that will interest and intrigue the reader.

## Paradise Memories

### Home of the Holchu

A little-known fact about Andaman and Nicobar Islands is that during World War II, the Japanese army had overrun the British here before launching towards Kohima. Japanese forces had grabbed Andaman and Nicobar Islands in March 1943, when they were at the peak of their power thrust. They carried out a number of developmental works to bring in self-sufficiency; however, their strict and harsh control resulted in rebellion by the locals. Subhas Chandra Bose visited in December 1943 and unfurled the 'tiranga' in Port Blair for the very first time. This was before the independence of the country in 1947. The islands were lovingly renamed 'Shaheed and Swaraj Dweep'. While the Andaman and Nicobar Islands passed into Indian hands on 15 August 1947, the airbase at Car Nicobar was formally taken over from the Royal Air Force in 1956 and established as Number 1 Staging Post.

Quite often, bullets would be dug out from ruined fortifications across the island. There are remnants of artillery guns and coastal batteries too. There was rumoured to be a well very close to where we stayed, where hundreds had been killed and thrown in by the Japanese. It was claimed by the locals that wails could still be heard in the night from this well. There was no way any local tribal or Holchu could be persuaded to venture anywhere near that area after sunset. Our evening, and sometimes night, walks often passed the place, but we never heard any wails. But, to be honest, in the loneliness of the island there was always a lingering worry about hearing them some night.

Kakana village and its beach, which were at one end of the runway, had some of the most beautiful sights on the entire island. The sea was too dangerous for swimming, but the crescent beach with its crashing waves made for a pretty sight to sit and watch under a coconut tree. A Holchu would never rest under a coconut tree; he knew what a falling coconut could do to you. It was a treat to see them climb a tree—faster than any other human. I guess that was one reason why they had such strong arms and legs. In fact, when the government introduced sports to the island on a wide scale, the Holchus did very well in those requiring strength and stamina. The women's cycling team were national champions at one time. Kakana village and its beach were completely destroyed in the tsunami of 2004. It never managed to regain even a fraction of its earlier beauty.

## Rich Tribal Diversity

The head of Car Nicobar island and the only cooperative person with an unpronounceable local name but an easier acronym, NHL, was a Muslim non-tribal. He was adopted by the tribal chieftain as a child. He in turn adopted Sam, a Holchu, as his prodigy. Among all the tribes of the Andaman, the Holchus have managed to thrive, modernize and yet keep their culture intact. Their villages are exceptionally clean and tidy. Their lineage is positively Mongoloid. On the other hand, tribes like Sentinelese, Jarawas and Onges in the Andamans are of Negroid descent. The Onges in Hut Bay on Little Andaman resemble pygmies. We often used to land there and interact because most outside teams such as parliamentary committees, anthropologists and academicians could only visit them. The local government had made houses on stilts for them, which they used to dutifully occupy during such visits. Once the visits were over, they preferred their ancient legacy of open skies and living in harmony with nature. Nobody dared to go anywhere near North Sentinel—in fact, no one has in recorded history. The Sentinelese are hostile to outside influences and are reputed to be cannibalistic. There was one person who used to go there alone in a boat with provisions. He would offload all the stuff on the beach and row out and wait. The Sentinelese would take the goods, leave tribal artefacts and other stuff on the beach, and retreat into the forest. The gentleman would row in, pick up the items and go back to Port Blair. Trust this person to be an enterprising Sikh gentleman!

### Unravelling a Mobike

I had moved my entire luggage to Car Nicobar (also called Carnic) on being posted there—the first person in the IAF's history to do so. It was foolish, but then I had no other place to dump it. So my motorcycle also came along. All this in a ship, and therefore, there was little to retrieve at the end. But the bike worked and the family enjoyed drives around the entire island—all 54 km of the perimeter road. A colleague borrowed it for a jaunt and unfortunately drove into a shallow pool, after which the engine jammed. There were no mechanics on the island. Pondy (actually Deshpande and inevitably nicknamed so) was by profession a pilot, but by nature a jack of all trades. He volunteered to repair it, and I agreed for want of a choice. A room, which was a hard-to-get commodity, was identified and vacated. Painstakingly, the bike was unravelled and the parts lined up in a sequenced trail on the floor so that getting it together would not be a problem. This took a month, after which another two weeks were spent cleaning the parts. Pondy was meticulous and did not trust us with helping out—so we were banned. However, even after a year, the bike though put together in one piece, never managed to fire. I took it along on being posted to Sarsawa after two years, and that is where she came back to life under a proper mechanic. Pilots should stick to flying!

### Carnic Capers

There was only one place safe for swimming on the entire island of Car Nicobar—Passa Beach. It was enclosed on one side by a right-angle turn that the island took and on the other by a huge coral reef. The water in between was clear with a shallow gradient for almost everyone—swimmers, non-swimmers and children—to enjoy the ocean. The reef allowed snorkelling; however, one had to take note of the razor-sharp edges of some of the corals.

At other places on the island, the Holchus used their boats, fitted with outriggers, to penetrate large waves for fishing and diving for exotic shells that fetched a good sum during the tourist season at Port Blair. I once went on such a ride. Despite my white-water rafting experience, this was truly thrilling. Once out in the ocean, the Holchus dived to depths of 10 metres or more to pluck out king shells and other prized corals. I did not dare to dive so deep into the wide ocean due to an inexplicable hidden fear, but I did indulge in snorkelling from the surface. I even caught sight of a huge manta ray for the first time in my life.

We once organized a para-sailing camp at the Carnic airbase for over a week, courtesy of a team from the AIR HQ adventure directorate in Delhi. My wife also took part and earned her certificate after five launches. The problem with Carnic runway was that it was too narrow, with hundreds of tall coconut trees aligned on either side. So, one had to be careful of prevailing winds lest one be blown into those menacing trees. All went well for almost 200 launches, till the station commander, Premi, decided that it was safe enough for him to try. Since he was a hard taskmaster, quite obviously a section of people did not particularly like him and came to watch hoping for some fun! And it happened. The winds changed as he got airborne and slowly, he drifted towards the coconut trees. The jeep picked up speed to get him higher and to avoid the trees, but now he was on top of them, just skimming the top branches and leaves. The jeep had only a few hundred metres of run left since the runway end was approaching fast. Just when we were losing hope and were assured of a skewered station commander, the winds changed and he drifted back to safety, just in time. It was quite disappointing for some of the onlookers!

## HAND-TO-MOUTH

The Holchus never grew, or at least never sold, any vegetables. Similarly, they fished only to sustain themselves. The end result was that nothing was available for mainlanders such as us. An-32 aircraft as twice-a-week couriers from Madras (now Chennai) were our lifelines. After every courier landing, the entire station would make a beeline for the plane to collect fresh vegetables, milk and everything else. The quality of servings at every home depended on whether the courier landed or not. For fish, we relied on our own Mi-8 weekly courier to Kamorta Island, from where gunny bags full of fish were bought and distributed to all families in the IAF camp. We all lived in temporary tin hutments or 'bashas' made of wood and hay. There were very few cemented structures. After I left, many solid structures, including a modern officer's mess, did come up overlooking the beautiful ocean. All were wiped out in a moment by the 2004 tsunami.

## Tsunami Travails

There were many heart-rending stories of what happened that fateful morning of 26 December 2004. It is believed that almost 20 per cent of the population of the Nicobar group of islands was wiped out. The IAF lost 119 personnel and family members. I know an officer who, along with his wife, had held on to their two little children dearly. When the deluge was over, their children were gone forever. Within days, the air force started operations and did 226 sorties over the next few weeks to evacuate 10,000 people. Mi-8s undertook rescue missions with gallant crew flying in their pyjamas and slippers since everything was lost. Barren Island, India's only active volcano, erupted after a few days because of seismic shocks. I remember flying over it and Narcondam (extinct volcano) in 1988. We had actually gone into the circular valley around the centre.

It was like a Shiva lingam—a central raised pyramid-like structure surrounded by a rim of hills. I still have beautiful photographs of the same. After the tsunami and its eruption, the geography is unrecognizable—all is gone. Such is nature's power.

## Action Stations

There were interesting operational interludes during the tenure at Carnic. Once, government officials at Port Blair, along with the navy and us, planned an elaborate operation to intercept gangs from abroad (Taiwan) that conducted illegal activities in the Little Andaman Island. It involved IAF Mi-8s slithering army troops down on the island at dawn, and naval ships and speedboats making surprise multiple entries with customs and police officials in tandem. A huge cache of arms, drugs, animal skins and other things was recovered. Estuarine crocodiles, an endangered salt-water species at Dugong Creek, were especially targeted for their skins by these thugs.

Another memorable operation was an SOS from a merchant ship during the thick of the 1989 monsoon. We launched in great earnest and located the adrift ship after about half an hour of search. There were low clouds and intermittent monsoon showers, so we were anyway at just 100 metres on the radio altimeter. The sea was dark and menacing, and the ship was bobbing around like a toy. It was only when we went lower for the rescue that we realized how big the waves were. My eyes, in trying to keep track of the ocean surface, shifted from looking down to the top of the front windscreen edges. Despite the best efforts of the gunner, it was impossible to stay steady over the ship. Fortunately, nobody was seen on the ship—maybe it was too dangerous to come out. But I salute helicopter pilots across the world who have successfully carried out such rescues—it is well-nigh impossible to do so unless fitted with better avionics and autopilot systems.

# DAKSHIN DRISHTIKONE

'THE SOUTHERN POINT of view' is about life in the relatively peaceful south India. As a military aviator, you often get posted to the south for training and instructional duties. In a chronological sense, this section covers this gamut of almost thirty years. It brings out the changing times, life and landscape.

From life as a rookie cadet at the academy and Helicopter Flying School to an instructor's trainer in Chennai, I have experienced some very diverse and unique events; for example, rescuing pilots who bale out from stricken aircraft. There are tales here of lessons in integrity and character-building, and even the first steps to improvisation or jugaad in the air. Some salubrious tales from the staff college near Ooty also bring out the rich diversity of our people, as well as the armed forces. And yes, there are amazingly unique tales too; for example, witnessing the deep divide among the Japanese and South Korean officers!

## Down Academy Alley

Growing up at the alma mater of IAF officers—the Air Force Academy (AFA)—is a unique experience. All branches are together under one roof and develop bonds that last an entire career. Just like the National Defence Academy alumni, whenever a gathering of coursemates takes place, most talk revolves around those days at the academy. Here are some of my recollections.

### Iq-bal the Majestic

The imposing cadets' mess at AFA had vintage aircraft such as Toofanis, Mysteres and Vampires placed all over, but the place of pride in the central garden next to the main portico was reserved for the MiG-21. It evoked endless dreams and visions in all our minds. Equally imposing was Iq-bal, meaning luck or fortune, a stuffed tiger in a glass case. It was a legacy of the maharaja days when the flying college was located at Jodhpur. It too evoked visions of joining No. 1 Squadron or Tigers as they are known all over the IAF. The flying curriculum kept us busy with very little time for leisure. Exams spoilt any chance of having fun in the initial two months. The only place cadets of the flying course would regularly make quick visits was to the temple complex, especially before really important flying tests that could result in you being shown the door. Of course, like the rest of humanity, God was quickly forgotten after the hurdle was crossed.

Coming back to Iq-bal. After a few months, once there was more time for reflection and 'velapanti', which is what you do when you have time and are bored, somebody queried as to why our tiger was named Iqbal. Bali, not known for being particularly insightful, got the answer first after he had a closer look. Iq-bal had, or at least what was visible, only one testicle! So 'one ball' became 'ek-ball' and took the majestic Punjabi evolution to Iq-bal. Or so Bali claimed!

### Camaraderie

IAF officers become accustomed to losing mates along the way in air crashes. Our very first one was John, who died in a Kiran crash within three months at AFA. It was a bolt from the blue and the first realization of how risky this business was. The crash took place around forenoon. After a pep talk, all of us were made to fly a sortie with our instructors in the afternoon. It was done to drive away the shock and fear, but also to help us learn an important lesson—the show must go on.

A few months later, we were having tea and snacks in the cafeteria, which had a grandstand view of the runway and flying operations, when two Kirans in close formation did a fly-past at low levels. And while we were watching, one suddenly dipped down . We later came to know that was because of an engine failure. The pilot, Golu, ejected and we saw it live, including his parachute landing far away. Before the chopper could come to pick him up, he had gathered his parachute, hitched a ride with a fuel truck on the way to AFA on the national highway, and was back with us—holding his coveted chute firmly (it's yours to keep after an ejection)!

As I mentioned earlier, training together with all branches of the IAF had its own perks. There was a strong and healthy rivalry between the courses, but also great camaraderie, especially against the common enemy—the instructional staff out to instil strict discipline. A flight lieutenant, Dash, in particular was a firebrand who was probably detailed to give our ground-course colleagues a hard time. One particular weekend he was really 'having' them with fall-in at awkward times, health runs, strenuous workouts and everything he had probably experienced himself as a cadet.

While going for dinner he caught Bali—yes, the same one who solved the Iq-bal mystery—for not being properly dressed. He gave him a harsh talking-to and sent him back to change.

Bali, who was going through some tough times in flying with frequent trips to the temple, was livid. After dinner, while strolling outside, he saw Dash's old scooter parked near the MiG with an even older helmet on it. Without further ado and despite our protests, he picked it up and, with a grand throw, flung it into the thicket next to the MiG. After this, we all made a run for it.

To cut a long story short, our ground-duty coursemates 'had' it for the next forty-eight hours. Dash's threat was clear—no respite till his helmet was returned. The entire weekend, normally a time of some rest, was consumed. We asked Bali to undo the problem. He empathized with our colleagues but refused to go anywhere near the MiG. By Sunday night, the grilling of our coursemates was getting intolerable. They had approached us for help while searching the entire mess and its surroundings. While many surprising things had been found, the helmet was still elusive—we could not tell them for fear of retribution. Duke and I gathered courage and finally, in the wee hours of Monday, retrieved the 'treasure', placed it squarely on Iq-bal's case and ran!

## Back in the Alley

As if on a pilgrimage such as the Kumbh, many of us come back to AFA after seven to eight years as qualified flying instructors (QFIs) to handle first-time rookie pilots. The first six months are a mix of stress, enthusiasm, trials and tribulations. First, you have to rough it out with your wife and kids in temporary rooms while waiting for a house. Second, timings of flying, briefings and debriefs, and other mundane tasks mean that you get very little time with the family. The temporary block was a three-storey building with multiple one-room set-ups. The staircase had a faulty railing—only one bar all along, through which a child could just walk through. And this did happen once—Mehta's two-year-old walked through and fell three storeys down. Miraculously, everything happened to save him. A cycle happened to be parked in exactly the right place, and its seat with springs cushioned the fall. The child fell on it in such a way that no damage was done!

Being a flying instructor is a unique experience—possibly the most profound personality developer in a pilot's career. It is a privilege to see raw rookies evolve into budding pilots in all aspects of skills, character and ethics. Every QFI develops his own distinct style of handling cadets. But I clearly remember one wise and old CO at Flying Instructor School remarking that a cadet learns to fly despite his instructor if he has the aptitude! There is so much truth in this singular observation—the only thing that really affects a rookie is the intent of his QFI. If that is honourable, all works out.

The bond between an instructor and his pupils is almost sacred and lifelong. You can rest assured that a pupil will only remember his instructor for the intent displayed. Also very true is the fact that an instructor's professional category may not truly reflect his success in producing or facilitating fine pilots. Patience and the willingness to allow mistakes are key. Some episodes involving flying by cadets are truly worth recollecting. When I was a cadet in AFA, we had two friends from Zambia—Sumwe and Makatale. Sumwe, all 6 feet 3 inches of him, could not fit in a Kiran and so went back. Makatale passed out with us but not before extracting some sweat and blood from the air traffic controllers at AFA. Once he came up on the radio in his heavily accented voice, 'Academy 136, my controls are not responding.' The entire tower panicked at the thought of a cadet in an uncontrolled aeroplane. The flight supervisor (an on-duty QFI) jumped up from the book he was reading and queried on the radio as to what his position was. Makatale said that he was on the dispersal on ground. Obviously he was doing his ground checks and was thoroughly annoyed at the wasted time and opportunity!

### Makatale's 'Moment'

Makatale had another memorable moment while training in India. We had all moved from AFA to Hakimpet. Makatale was training on a Kiran aircraft in Fighter Training Wing (FTW) with his instructor, when the engine suddenly gave up over a very rocky and large-boulder-infested area. Both ejected and landed safely; however, the instructor had a slight ankle sprain. Makatale was absolutely hale and hearty. Within no time, a rescue chopper landed alongside. The doctor and attendant appeared with a stretcher. A debate then ensued about who to evacuate first. Makatale insisted on his instructor being taken away first, while the doctor's priority was the foreigner since neither of them were seriously injured. Finally, the doctor prevailed and a fully fit Makatale was made to lie on the stretcher to be taken to the running chopper. On the way, the stretcher's fabric gave away and down came Makatale. Now he had a serious back injury. A second stretcher, a quick chopper ride to the hospital and good care got him back into the cockpit after a month. Makatale finally understood Murphy's Law in totality!

Another case was of a naval aviator, Pillai, who was out on a first solo in the sector, which meant away from the runway. After coming overhead, he claimed that he was seeing a black runway (the one at AFA was white). Also, he said that the aircraft seemed to be touching the runway at Hakimpet (further away) in his turns to do a rectangular pattern for landing. All eyes went up to the skies, but there was no Pillai around. On a complaint from nearby airfields, Pillai was finally spotted. He had misread all his instruments—height of 2,000 instead of the 12,000 feet that he was at, and a speed of 150 knots instead of the 250 knots that he was pelting at.

Essentially, he was rocketing around the whole place without a clue. He was finally escorted down by a QFI in another Kiran after much catching up. Pillai never managed to make it as an aviator, but it seems he did very well as a submariner! That's destiny for you.

**Honesty Pays!**

As trainees (just commissioned officers) at HTS and FTW, we used to stay in an old and far-flung mess. No duty officer or instructor would bother to check on us—thus ensuring complete freedom! All of us had bicycles to pedal to work. Incidentally, most of us could not afford to buy a motorcycle. Also, because of an accident in the previous course, a couple of our coursemates whose parents could gift them bikes were effectively dissuaded from doing so.

One hot afternoon, my coursemate Neat* and I were riding down in our khaki uniforms. Neat had tried all forms of intoxication, including the favourite village brew 'tadi', or toddy. Seeing a woman selling the same in old beer bottles, he stopped. I wasn't keen to try any local stuff, but he persisted since no one was around. Curiosity got the better of prudence, and I took a swig. It was so horrible that I spat it out immediately. Neat polished off both the bottles without further ado.

Little did we know that a sergeant in civil clothes had witnessed the scene and reported it to the station adjutant. The next day, scheduled for afternoon-flying, I reached HTS by 10 a.m. to attend classes. It was puzzling to not hear the familiar drone of helicopters. I got my answer in a fall-in of the whole trainee course of HTS outside the CO's office. I apologetically joined in late with a good glare from the chief ground instructor. He was bawling out that there would be no further flying till the two officers who had tadi

---

* Name changed.

owned up. Among our coursemates were around thirty captains and majors of the Indian Army. The chief ground instructor gave a last and final call. I immediately stepped out and owned up, hoping Neat would too. The next fifteen minutes were used by every available instructor to threaten, warn, cajole and try everything else on me to reveal the 'other'. I refused to tattle and said that I was taking responsibility for what I did, but would not take any other name.

Finally, I was marched up to the CO after he had been briefed. Those were times when COs were hardly seen, except for a final suspension check or a trophy check in flying—both momentous occasions. He was a diminutive man but displayed great strength and control. He point-blank asked me whether I was willing to be suspended for not revealing the other officer's name. I had realized that if Neat's name came out now, his goose would surely be cooked. I kept quiet. On being asked why I was not revealing the name, I gave a reply invoking the NDA spirit of camaraderie. That saved me. The CO closed the case and ordered my instructor, the CFI, to give me a bottle of good whisky, advising him to take care of my good spirits! While all coursemates, including Neat, enjoyed the expensive whisky, the larger lesson of 'honesty pays' was not lost on them.

There is more to this thread. Some twenty-five years later, Neat was commanding a frontline base in an area where counter-insurgency operations were in full swing. While there was no need for it, he went as a co-pilot on one of the 'hot' missions. To cut a long story short, he agreed to the army's urgent request to carry excess load from a forward helipad. Despite objections from the young captain (a wing commander), he insisted on helping out with the take-off. The helicopter crashed but, fortunately, nobody died or was injured much.

With a good career ahead of him, Neat first tried to coerce the captain to take full blame, and then officially denied involvement in the inquiry that followed. However, senior officers at the Command HQ were not fooled and the truth did come out. Neat's future was sealed and a clear-cut message was sent out that errors and mistakes, and accountability, are not the domain of junior ranks only.

Sometimes I wonder if coming out with the truth as a better and safer option is really so difficult to fathom. I have heard many colleagues talk about traits displayed as cadets (under heavy stress and distress) that are innate and come out when the going gets tough. It seemed to be true in this case, and many other cases that one witnessed in the services.

## Tambaram Tamasha

The Flying Instructors School (FIS) is the Mecca for flying instructors. Except for the sweltering and humid conditions most of the time, the work is fast-paced and satisfying. The best of IAF personnel come to become QFIs, and it is a learning experience for all. Mutuals or sorties done amongst student officers are the best because of the freedom and competitiveness attached. Actually, one learns far more during these than the regular ones with staff. As staff, life was easier handling experienced students unlike at the academy. It was also fun to jump from a piston-propeller HPT-32 to a jet (Kiran) cockpit between sorties. And after four sorties, to come back and take classes for a very discerning and questioning lot of pilots was gratifying, to say the least. Being the junior most staff, quite logically, most of the unwanted jobs such as taking tough classes, tea club management, among others, fell on my shoulders. Our CO, Murli, was a rare category-AQFI, and a great human being. He ensured all of us got our commercial licences, besides ensuring thorough professional output at FIS. His belief was that it gave officers a 'spine' to do their duty.

Chennai used to be threatened sometimes with a rare cyclone, especially in the autumn, which, instead of re-curving northwards, headed straight for it. But this happened once in a decade or so. An annual ritual was to get to a high-alert level with the meteorology department tracking these storms—all ready to quickly make a run to Bangalore with our planes. In my first year in 1993, we picked up all our thirty-plus aircraft and ferried to Bangalore. We spent two days watching movies, including a just-released *The Silence of the Lambs*, and generally unwound. It was back to FIS humdrum after two days since the cyclone, as usual, missed Chennai. The next year, after dutifully checking with and an assurance from the meteorology guys, Murli took the decision of not ferrying out. That night, the cyclone hit us squarely. I remember going out to my garden around 2 a.m. when the eye with its eerie calm passed by. Ferocious winds and rain brought down half the trees and poles in Tambaram, but all hangars with their aeroplanes survived the night. Some of them were pre-Independence vintage—just goes to show the quality of construction of that era.

### Money-Mani

Mani was a rickshaw-puller who by pure chance happened to ferry my wife, Sheel, a couple of times to the railway station on her frequent trips to Nalli and Kumaran—famous saree stores—mainly for window shopping. He was a simple man who had lost one eye as a child. His sincerity and honesty were endearing, and therefore, he ended up doubling as our gardener too. It is amazing what high morals can be ingrained in someone so poor. He wept inconsolably when we were posted out, but I made sure he was recommended to another officer who was posted in. In a year, he became the personal help of a student, and later staff, who had come all the way from the USA. Once again, he impressed him so much that he offered to take him to the US. But Mani, being who he was, declined. He was well rewarded and, the last I heard, had bought a couple of motorized rickshaws and was doing well as an entrepreneur.

### Teesta the Tree!

My last fond memory of Tambaram is of my daughter taking her first steps into an air force school. She did not cry on the first day, unlike my son a few years later, and took to school like a fish to water. So when the fancy-dress competition for the annual day came along, she was looking forward to dressing up as a little fairy with a cute poem all memorized. In our busy schedule, both my wife and I completely forgot about the dress till reminded by Teesta the night before the competition. It was too late to do anything. I conned her into becoming a tree with a 'save the trees' message (this was in 1993). After some crying and promises of presents later, she agreed and stood first in the competition for giving out a visionary message for the future! Incidentally, I named her Teesta after the famous river in Sikkim and Bengal, the first one I crossed in my helicopter as a pilot officer.

## Alma Mater—Chopper Men

I use the word 'men' with purpose and clarity. The diverse interaction and a need to operate absolutely independently on the run brings maturity and wisdom to us earlier than others. Our alma mater, the HTS, is the start point of this journey. The school has modernized and grown over the years, in keeping with the pace of growth of the service as such. However, even today, the gurukul concept is still followed. An instructor has ownership of a bunch of just-commissioned officers, which defines his duty. Similarly, the trainees, or 'chelas', look up to him for unadulterated honourable intent and attention. Face-to-face briefs, debriefs and 'chai pe charcha' or discussions over a cup of tea are still the backbone of life in HTS.

As a CO, I had taken it upon myself to revamp an almost four decade-old unchanged syllabus. I must admit that Wing Commander Singdeo, a rare category-A flying instructor, who had retired in the 1980s, was instrumental in pushing me in that direction. He had been advocating it for decades and only gave up after he retired. I studied the flying syllabi of at least ten different modern and some not-so-modern air forces. The logic of change being needed was clear.

The first step was to disturb the equilibrium or comfort zones that HTS had gone into. I prepared a controversial paper that did precisely this—irked most and irritated many. But it set a cat among the pigeons with healthy, and sometimes unhealthy, debates and discussions. Newer manoeuvres and exercises that met the demands of modern battlefields were tried out. At the end of six months, a syllabus completely different from the one followed over decades, and also quite evolved from what I had envisaged originally, was ready to be fought over with the outside world.

Numerous presentations and debates later with the Command and Air HQ, I was ready to present it to my chief and vice-chief. The chief, a helicopter pilot himself, was convinced by the second presentation, but the vice-chief was still sceptical. While giving his approval, the CAS remarked, 'What the hell were we doing so far?' The vice-chief murmured something about the guys hopefully knowing what they were doing in terms of safety. The new programme was lapped up by all, especially trainees, because of the better challenges to build their skills and situational awareness. Over the years, it has shown great results in skill-building. Imagine my surprise and happiness when, during a reunion party some years later at HTS, some young instructors came up to me and went on to explain a modern way of training being followed. I did not want to dampen their enthusiasm and listened in mock awe about the huge changes happening. The trials, travails and tribulations of the effort will always remain a deeply satisfying personal memory.

### Games People Play!

I had just taken over command of HTS when I was made the task force in charge of a parachuting event of the military world games to be held in Hyderabad in 2007. I had not fully got into the groove of running HTS. The event was big, with militaries from all over the world participating. Air Force Station, Hakimpet, was given the whole responsibility of the competition, which is a unique military event.

I went over the draft plan of action that the station had been working on. It was poorly done and the inherent inefficiencies could not have handled the more than 3,000 jumps planned. The AOC and I crossed swords on the issue. Finally, I was called to Air HQ to present my logic, which was entirely agreed to. The event thereafter went flawlessly. It was amazing to watch the accuracies achieved by jumpers on that small circle of cushions. This included women jumpers from some militaries; in fact, the best score was by a lady from Austria. The president of the commission presented me a plaque acknowledging the completion of 3,000 jumps for the first time ever. Hakimpet had put its heart into making the event a success. It was a proud moment, but I could never make up with my AOC till he left on posting. I am still trying to figure out what went wrong.

## Salubrious Wellington

I came across the word 'salubrious' for the first time when we arrived at Conoor to do the staff course. Within a year, the importance of the word was well ingrained. It was heaven on earth—climate, locale, facilities and bandobast (arrangements), and the people. It was an ever-learning year with young officers from all three services putting their minds together at a still impressionable age. The air wing's curriculum was rated fifth in terms of degree of difficulty—after the army, navy, KV School and Holy Angels School, where our children studied. Be that as it may, at the end of the course, everyone was convinced that true assimilation and application came best in the air wing—maybe the balance between learning and competition was just right.

A much-awaited event was the monthly hikes to explore various parts of Coorg. Extremely well organized with expert army bandobast, they were looked forward to by both parents and children. When we first moved into the ground floor house on top of Gurkha Hill, the first three days went in toiling hard to set up the house sans any help. We noticed our neighbour's house (an army officer) already ready and lit up. So we went there on the third evening after our arrival. Imagine our surprise at being told by the two sahayaks that the officer and his wife would arrive only the next day. They had set up the house all by themselves. It was one of the rare times Sheel wished I had joined the army instead.

I should talk more about Sheel. I had tried to teach her how to drive a car at Tambaram. In exasperation at my incompetence and impatience, she had walked out of the car, never to allow me to instruct her again. It was a shock—after all; I was a category-A instructor at FIS! However, she got back at me in Wellington. I was out for a ten-day trip, all in a train, to visit various industrial demonstrations across southern India. When I came back, she suggested we go to the shopping arcade all the way down the hill and then up towards the college. I moved towards the car, but before I could, she had occupied the driver's seat. And to my surprise, she drove perfectly all the way and back. There was an old driver in Wellington who was a favourite with the ladies for learning how to drive. An old man's patience and wisdom perfectly matched their learning graph!

## The Ten Commandments

The commandant, General Baldev, was another wise old man. He had started a course for ladies, full of interaction with diverse speakers and experts from various walks of life. It was topped by a final lecture by the general himself on 'Baldev's ten commandments'. While all were pearls of wisdom, two were outstanding and have withstood the test of time. The first was that whenever one door shuts, another one opens—obviously alluding to opportunities in one's career. The other was to respect and accept the element of 'kismat' or fate. At the end of all our efforts, things may not work out the way one designed or envisaged. I think deep down, Gen. Baldev knew that burning ambitions were driven on both wheels—the officer and his better half.

## History Divides

Among our staff college coursemates in the air wing were a British RAF navigator, a Japanese and a South Korean, both pilots. I was close to John, the RAF officer, and we used to indulge in a lot of banter. After almost six months, the Korean officer came up to me and asked me a very perplexing question. 'Why are you so close to a British national?' he asked. 'Why not?' I replied. To my amazement, he reminded me of the 200-year-old British rule over India.

And then he said something more amazing—had I ever seen him being so friendly with the Japanese officer? The Japanese travesty in Korea around WWII could never be forgiven. I was stumped for an answer—history runs really deep in East Asia.

### The Interview

Our chief instructor (CI) was an erudite and eloquent gentleman. A very suave professional, he must have liked what I brought to the table during debates and discussions with the army and navy officers, since I had extensive experience working with both. So he must have thought it right to call me for a tête-à-tête on finer grooming issues. His point revolved around sports that I indulged in. I had been playing basketball and volleyball, and our division had won both championships. I even got something akin to a Blue in NDA—I think a Cravat. He asked me about golf, and my straight shot from the hip was that it was for old men. He seemed to be taken aback and I immediately realized that I had put my foot in my mouth. Anyway, he dropped the subject and moved on. I did not pick up golf even in Hindon, where my house was just a few yards from the course. And the irony is that when I did learn, I grew very fond of the game. I still regret the loss of opportunity at Wellington and Hindon. It is a great game where the primary opposition is yourself—it's mainly about over-ambition and over-stretching beyond your capability. There cannot be a better way to see through a person and get to his real character than indulging in a round of golf. A great game indeed—the CI was right.

# MADHYAM MELA

THE LITERAL TRANSLATION of this title is 'Central Circus'! It covers many changes that took place over the decades while I was posted and flying in the central part of India—chiefly in Uttar Pradesh (UP).

This section includes tales about pioneering superhighways as runways for fighter-jet operations to interacting with civilian leaders. As an air force examiner, one travelled across the entire country from the base at Hindon. It was a perfect bird's-eye view of how changes were taking place, not only in the IAF but across the country. It also brought out the evolving issues in an officer's conduct—social graces, effects of social media and the many new disruptions to our social fabric. It sure is a fast-changing world!

## Eagle Eyes—AEB

The aircrew examining board (AEB) at Hindon is a filter that ensures the highest standards of knowledge, professionalism and aviation skills among pilots. I reached there with my family from staff college, not realizing what awaited us.

## Better to Be an Examinee

All helicopter squadrons had to be visited at least twice a year, and training establishments up to four times. Each visit lasted from Monday to Saturday, which is why we were colloquially referred to as weekend husbands. A chopper examiner had a lot on his plate—at least thirty to forty day and night sorties, double that number of detailed briefings and debriefs, meetings with the CO and other supervisors—the list was endless. By the time I got posted out after three years, I had actually done 136 visits. There was no other job in the IAF that gave you a better pulse of operations in field units. I flew with every helicopter pilot of the fleet in every sector of operations. One did float operations over sea, deck landing, off-shore oil rig landing, special operations, glacier landing and many others. The flip side was that you had to be good in terms of knowledge and skills, because quite often you demonstrated or were requested to show ideal manoeuvres in the air—a difficult talk to walk. Given the various machines that one flew, this was really a tall order.

## Damu's Eulogy

Our CO was the late Damu. With a heart of gold and courage of conviction that I have yet to see again, he was a role model for all examiners. Unfortunately, he and another examiner, Roychow, met an untimely death in a chopper crash. They were attempting to reach a base when sudden thick fog engulfed them. It was a miserable week for the AEB fraternity. Mrs Damu settled in Bangalore with her children, while Mrs Roychow continued in Delhi. We were in touch with them for a long time. The IAF has an excellent support system in these cases, but the real strength comes from the friends one makes in service.

### Not So Mighty

Examining the air force also threw up some surprises, especially in terms of how innovative people could be to pass the ground test. Two cases in point have great humour in them. The first was in Sarsawa where we had gone to examine two very operational squadrons. One had its full complement of fifteen pilots, while Mighty Armours (my ex-unit) had only five. All the papers were in my briefcase, which had a number lock. Since we were to fly a few sorties before the written exam, I decided to take my briefcase along in the Mi-17. Tipsy, who was the flight commander and my old chum from the Aizawl days, offered his locked cupboard. With the cupboard keys in my pocket and Tipsy going with me for the sortie, I was completely at ease and reassured. During the test, while I was invigilating and Bads (my co-examiner) was checking the first submitted set of papers, disaster loomed. Bads took me aside and said that all five papers of one unit (you know which one) had scored 99 per cent or more. The next morning, we declared a retest for the five pilots, against which the CO and all pilots took up cudgels. When they were politely explained the fifty ways that we could fail them, including a viva, they relented. None of them managed to upgrade and only confirmed their earlier abilities. Finally, Tipsy let out the secret. It had to do with the duplicate keys of his cupboard, the easy picking of the number lock when put against a bright light, the quick photocopying, and most importantly, the solemn promise among them to score only what was required for an upgrade. But unlike the fabled honour among thieves, each tried to achieve a lifetime record!

### Dolly's Dunk

The second instance happened in AEB itself. Dolly was a chopper pilot known across the fleet for the use of the English language (or rather misuse). No gathering could be complete without him regaling us with some of his anecdotes. He somehow became a favourite of our new CO, Singhi. The only thing stopping Dolly from commanding a squadron was the absence of a 'Master-Green'—the highest instrument rating. Now, Dolly could never clear a paper, let alone do well. So, Singhi called Bads and expressed his desire for Dolly to pass. He, in fact, asked for a copy of the paper to be administered. A CO is a CO, and since this was done in the presence of another senior groupie from the chopper fleet, Bads had no choice. The test was scheduled for Monday morning, and Singhi was flying to Gorakhpur at 9 a.m. We delayed the paper till after he left and then Bads gave Dolly the most difficult set of papers that we had. Dolly wanted to leave, but we invoked clauses that could keep him out of the cockpit forever. His paper was marked and failed—all in red un-erasable ink and preserved. With a firm warning, he was shown the door. Singhi never got back to Bads about this; however, Bads never made it to the next rank in all his three attempts and took premature retirement. He was a fine and honest officer with a rare blend of vision and forthrightness. He is now doing well, after getting into trouble over similar integrity issues, for which he took successful legal recourse.

## Andaz-e-Lucknow

### A Happening Highway

A highpoint of my tenure as AOC at Surya, or the army's central command, was the construction of an aircraft landing strip on the then upcoming Agra–Lucknow Expressway. Many air forces use specially built highways for fighter aircraft operations to obviate closure of operations when regular airfields take a hit. But it had never been tried out in India. In 2015, one landing was carried out on the expressway between Delhi and Agra. This was just a one-off exercise, full of risks because of the divider in the centre of the road. However, it did catch everybody's attention.

My C-in-C urged me to follow up on this with a proper landing strip being built on the expressway coming up between Agra and Lucknow. The first heart and mind to be convinced was the young and dynamic chief minister of UP. Akhilesh Yadav not only turned out to be a large-hearted man but also a visionary politician. He was willing but was sceptical of his cabinet and bureaucrats. A detailed briefing on PowerPoint was carried out for both sides. Invoking China and the strategic importance of such an asset in terms of not only war but also disaster management seemed to convince them. There were still many hiccups over the next six months, including total costs that were to be incurred by the state. The funniest part was that a basic requirement of a 3-km-long straight stretch without bridges or pylons could not be met on the entire 300-plus km proposed road. I checked this out myself over each patch. Essentially, the road curved at every possible 'politically right' corner!

Finally, a stretch of just about 3 km was located 60 km from Lucknow. The relocation of a high-tension feeder line to about 3 km away required additional sanction from the government. Another meeting with the CM ensured it, but there was another and bigger problem waiting. The stretch was divided between contracts awarded to two different companies, which could have caused problems in design and quality control. It took quite an effort to change this but finally, Larsen & Toubro, a reputed company, got going on the full stretch. My team and I visited the site regularly for inspection and problem-solving, along with the main government supervisors Uttar Pradesh Expressways Industrial Development Authority (UPEIDA).

The chairman of UPEIDA was Navneet Sehgal, a dynamic officer who could really make things happen. Quick decision-making and flexibility were his core qualities. He should get a major credit for understanding all our complex requirements and standards. However, when the expressway was about to be inaugurated by the CM in November 2016, there was an unfortunate accident. Two days prior to the event, I had landed my chopper on the highway, while Sehgal had come in his official Ambassador car. He barely used to fit in it because of his height—6 feet and 4 inches. We had a long and detailed meeting with all stakeholders at the site, along with low passes being carried out by fighter aircraft as a trial for the main event. We finished around 2 p.m., and Sehgal offered me a lift in his car. My chopper had arrived by then. However, I couldn't reciprocate since we were not allowed to carry civilians. When I landed in Lucknow, the pilots informed me about some garbled radio transmission of a casualty evacuation.

By evening, it was all on TV. On the highway, assuming no traffic since it had not been declared open, Sehgal's driver zipped through a small dust cloud raised by the dust at a work site. That's when a maverick, who had managed to get his car up for a fun ride, happened to be in the same patch at precisely the same time, speeding in the opposite direction. The cars collided. While the driver died on the spot, Sehgal was trapped inside. His skull had serious injuries, and with multiple fractures, he was bleeding profusely. None of the locals present knew how to help. But like in all such preordained events, a miracle happened. Our specialist crash crew that handled aircraft crashes and prised out pilots from similar situations was also returning from the site. In fact, Sehgal's car had overtaken them just five minutes back. They had the skills and the equipment, and they immediately swung into action. Unfortunately, there was no doctor or medico available. But they took all care since they were fully trained in first aid. Sehgal's skull was bound up by handkerchiefs and he was rushed to the nearest hospital. A long ordeal of recovery followed, but now Sehgal is back in his chair and getting back to normal life fast. We missed him during the inauguration where eighteen landings and take-offs by SU-30s and Mirages was a first, with nationwide coverage by all media outlets. While there was some inevitable political hue, the IAF's prowess and professional skills were amply displayed.

### Muawaza Maanyata

Akhilesh Yadav's large-heartedness towards the armed forces was displayed in another interesting case. One HAL-built helicopter of the IAF had crashed near Lucknow in 2014. Seven people had perished, including two pilots and five ground crew. The captain was TNB, who had served under me in HTS and done a wonderful job during the Kurnool floods of 2009. Air Marshal Gill, on taking over as C-in-C, had very aptly observed a minute's silence to pay homage. He also requested me to approach the state government for monetary compensation since some of the widows or old parents of the deceased were from really poor backgrounds. I met the CM, and it did not take much to convince him. It, however, took almost a year of chasing various ministries to persistently push the file. The problem was that none of the deceased were from UP and, therefore, not covered under the state scheme. It was something that even the CM could not dislodge. But all credit to him that he dug into his own CM funds, over which he had some discretionary powers, to grant Rs 20 lakh to each family. At a befitting function with the CM, the chief of the air staff and the AOC-in-C, cheques were presented to all the families and citations read. Most family members had tears of gratitude in their eyes at the recognition accorded.

### Surya Shine

The army commander in Lucknow was General Rajan Bakshi. We went all the way back to our collaboration in Leh, where he was the corps commander and I the AOC of the airbase. Those wonderful stories have figured in a previous section of this book. However, it was a pleasant surprise to meet him once again, in Surya Command. Always generous and positive about airpower and jointness, he used to receive me warmly with a 'jhappi', or a warm hug—which never stopped surprising the generally stiff-upper-lip military echelons. Lucknow had more than twenty two-star generals, and we had a monthly reunion called the 2-Star Club, which was very well attended. Besides giving 'voice', aka karaoke, and reverting to batchmates' reunion antics, a lot of work was done at these informal gatherings.

### General Negi

After General Bakshi, General Negi took over as army commander in Lucknow. In Leh, too, he had taken over from General Bakshi as corps commander. I was on wonderful terms with him too. Negi was a bachelor who devoted his entire time and focus to the army and the nation. He was both admired and feared for his honesty and sense of justice. I had personally witnessed his courage of conviction in the stand-offs against the Chinese army in Ladakh, especially the one in Chumar. A great believer of jointness in the services in general, and air power in particular, he walked the talk on issues that affected them.

I remember accompanying members of the Central Pay Commission headed by retired Justice Mathur for a five-day trip to Ladakh. I was in Lucknow then and had been especially deputed by Air HQ. The itinerary was well planned to bring home the highest degree of difficulty and risks taken by air warriors and soldiers in this area. It covered Leh, Thoise, Kargil, Daulat Beg Oldie and, of course, the Siachen Glacier. All commission members were completely bowled over and moved by what they saw and experienced. Justice Mathur's parting words to Negi and me were: 'Whatever happens, the Siachen allowance will be the highest of the land.' General Negi still quotes that memorable effort at every occasion he gets to espouse jointness.

## Times Are a-Changin'

### A Techno-society: Boon or Bane?

My family's first wireless telephone experience was a large wireless local loop handset (WLL) that had a limited range and was as big as a traditional hand-held telephone (cordless). This was way back in 2003, just before I left for the Congo on a UN peacekeeping mission. In this conflict zone, I came across my first mobile phone set. Vodafone, a South African company, dominated the entire country's coverage. Mobile telephony was the only means of communication, and it was very effectively used by rebels, government soldiers and the UN.

Some major tactical battles between rival militia were fought purely on mobile communication. Let me explain. A marauding militia group approaching a rival camp was assessed by its numbers and weapons, varying from tens to hundreds. Spotters at exclusively chosen places provided early warnings by mobiles to the main camp. Here, a decision was taken to hold or flee—mostly the latter if the numbers were even marginally more. So most times, no actual fighting took place, but bullets were fired to celebrate victory. Only the local populace suffered. Even during the fall of Bukavu in

2003, no real fighting took place. But the entire financial capital of North Kivu was plundered and pillaged at will. Fiery exchanges mostly happened on mobiles or walkie-talkies.

Yet the same mobile connectivity was effectively used by the UN to build awareness and receptivity around numerous public programmes. The other important medium was FM radio. We could very well gather that music and rhythm was in the locals' blood, and if messages could ride this, the public would be ready to sway. It was strange to find a country as large as the whole of Europe with only a hundred-odd kilometres of tarred roads. The other links, the few that existed, were mud tracks that were almost non-negotiable in the incessant rains. And yet, the DRC probably had the highest density of advance landing strips—bare grounds fit only for light aircraft that merrily ferried out precious metals and coltan. It was a great exploitative model that filled the pockets of the unscrupulous elite while impoverishing the public over decades. It was almost as if King Leopold's inhuman means were replaced by others, albeit more tech-savvy.

In the twentieth century, we were used to long-drawn-out evolutionary changes that took decades in the IAF. This, despite being a more technology-driven service in comparison. However, mobiles and apps have changed the game—at least socially. WhatsApp came about in the IAF around 2013—a great example of its innovative use was in Operation Rahat—the relief operations in Uttarakhand. Most of us, except some of the younger lot, were not even aware of it. But in just five years, at least my family can't imagine what life was like in the non-social-media days! All of us prioritize virtual connectivity over real connect.

Today, most crimes are solved thanks to CCTV coverage, mobile tracking or uncovering digital transactions. Although these may have enabled and empowered criminals and petty thieves, the other side of the coin is that evidence-gathering and tracking has become easier for the police. I witnessed and arrived at a similar conclusion during my tenure as a Senior Officer Administration (SOA). Almost everything, except for flying operations and maintenance of aircraft and systems, fell on the SOA's plate—meaning all good and dirty tasks. It was easier to synergize the legal and policing arms since both came under the SOA.

I firmly believe that the armed forces are but a reflection of society at large, albeit with more self-discipline—maybe due to faster and surer accountability. And yet, the motives for misdemeanour remain essentially the same—greed, low morals and a patriarchal mindset. Since the chances of getting caught and 'fixed' are much higher than Civvy Street, the crime rates are much lower. The key to deterrence then was increasing the chances of getting caught—CCTVs, encouraging whistle-blowers, protecting ethically correct behaviour, etc. But the most important was to 'walk the talk' yourself. I was fortunate to have Zapo as my commander in Central Air Command—a man of ethics and integrity. Down the line it was easier to execute—it was just a matter of personal choice. A case in point was the exemplary punishment to those violating Vishaka norms under the new sexual harassment at the workplace law. Another interesting case was a person blackmailing a girl over some explicit mobile pictures. A well-thought-out trap, some cyber expertise and other measures ensured that a damsel was freed and justice was served. Imagine how much time these cases would have taken outside the armed forces. Another important issue was an effective programme to sensitize people, especially those very gullible, against unscrupulous Ponzi schemes and other frauds. Case studies and open discussion forums were the most effective methods to do so.

## 'Culture Shock'

Air Marshal Inamdar's booklet titled 'Towards Fewer Faux Pas and Gaffes' was very handy when we were young officers. It was all about being groomed into officers who were chivalrous, courteous, disciplined and embodied social finesse. It was recommended to youngsters by senior officers; in fact, I have heard numerous talks based on the booklet over the years at many bases. Simple tips on how to guide a senior inspecting officer around or how to ask a lady for a dance at a party were a great help to those being initiated into a social set-up that was moulded by a strong British legacy. But to be very honest, even in our young days, we did find some of it irrelevant and superfluous—little realizing the need for defined social behaviour norms in such a structured and hierarchical organization as ours.

At officer mess parties, it was a done thing to walk up to a lady and ask her for a dance. There was a protocol of how to lead her, as also how to dance with grace, keeping up with her dance steps (and capabilities). The music inevitably started with ghazals or Western pop numbers (mainly oldies) with no question of vulgar or 'embarrassing' numbers. You got a regular debrief on your social conduct—or lack of it—by the flight commander the next day. All this has changed now. The music is much louder—in every conceivable way. Bollywood hits—dominated by Punjabi colours and hues—are the start and end of all parties. Numbers that may be slightly uncomfortable to older generations are played out loud and danced to with passion. An even more surprising development is the disappearance of the tradition of asking a lady for a dance. It is quite normal to see groups of ladies or men dancing vigorously but separately. 'Paisa vasool', or getting your money's worth, seems to be the new mantra. But quite clearly, parties are being enjoyed more to let your hair down than as opportunities for social interaction. In fact, that part is done more on Facebook and WhatsApp!

I think it was easier to manage youngsters' josh and energy as COs earlier than it is in an age of the internet. A simple lights-out time monitoring could ensure enough sleep before the next day's work or flying. Today, without the option of jamming the net, how much time is spent on Facebook, WhatsApp and the like is anybody's guess. Connectivity of the constant kind comes at a heavy price. 'No news is good news', an old adage, allowed peace of mind. The new 'constant connect' brings in a myriad of constant worries, interference, micromanagement and other such ills.

But then it has also ensured far greater transparency and accountability as a whole. Gone are the days when leaders or senior officers at any level could get away with acts that were downright unethical. Any person today has several avenues to put forth an issue for redressal. This has increased the workload to handle and process this, but it has forced leaders to be more accountable.

## What's in a Name?

The legacy of short and easy nicknames comes from the need for quick radio transmissions in air combat. Long-winded names, resulting in longer time to communicate, may result in disastrous consequences. As such, while flying combat missions, each pilot of a squadron gets a call sign out of a sequenced series typical of each combat squadron. So, you could find the CO being called 'Scotch', and so on, and the youngest pilot being called 'Soda' or something. Some squadrons have names based on predatory animals or venomous snakes, and some transport aircraft squadrons have named themselves after beasts of burdens such as camels, oxen and the like.

## Nicking Names

Nicknaming seems to have its own logic—with a clear method in the madness. For example, in the IAF, all Deshpandes become Pondy or Deshu depending on their general demeanour or penchant for mischief. A serious or reticent fellow is obviously Deshu. Most Ahluwalias are rounded off as Ahlus. Pudding was an exception to this, probably because of his penchant for sweeter stuff that overrode traditional naming. All Shankers got shortened to Shanks, as did many others like Chow and Dixie (Chowdhary, Dikshit). In a squadron with two Asthanas, one was named Asty and the other Nasty—quite obviously reflecting their personae. Some popular nicknames transcended religion. A Sam could be a Sindhi Samtani or a Christian Samuel, or even a Hindu Sammadar. Some names were purely based on personality traits. Zapo was a shortened version of someone who zapped you with his out-of-the-box thinking or ideas, while his real name was Sinha. Somehow I escaped getting a nickname. 'Isser' was short and easy on the tongue—there was no need to corrupt it!

## A Tribute to Fallen Comrades

I've recounted stories earlier around the Walong War Memorial. It is now a befitting tribute to soldiers and air warriors of yesteryears, especially the 1962 War (with permanent inauguration plaques!). The IAF has been late in catching up with war memorials. The Longewala episode of 1971 was hardly ever paid tribute to except in writings or speeches. A beginning was made with a small memorial within Jaisalmer airbase. But now there is a befitting memorial near Longewala, complete with Pakistani tanks and Hunters that butchered them on that famous morning in December 1971. At Allahabad, a new war memorial was inaugurated in 2017 with another Hunter in the backdrop. Aircraft from Central Air Command took part on both the eastern and western sectors. The Tangail Airdrop operation involved many bases such as Darbhanga, Bihta and Allahabad.

## Bamrauli Banter

Allahabad, now Prayagraj, has a long history linked to the very first aviation activities in India. In 1923, the first air mail was operated between Bamrauli and Naini across the mighty Ganges. The legacy buildings housing the air traffic control and passenger terminal still stand today. Most of the current air force set-up was a guava orchard belonging to one Mir Ali, an erstwhile nawab. Across Sangam is another abandoned base of Phaphamau. It saw considerable action during World War II with many aeroplanes taking part in 'over the hump' operations against the Japanese army. After almost sixty years, we reclaimed the base, building a concrete wall around it. In 2018, we also landed a C-130J Hercules there while simulating a mass casualty evacuation.

# EPILOGUE

## A Tribute to Those Magnificent Machines

THE INDIAN HELICOPTER story began on 10 March 1954 with the formation of the 104 Helicopter Unit (HU) in New Delhi, equipped with Sikorsky S-55s. The pioneers were Mazumdar and Todd who started this glorious story. In the first year itself, helicopters came into the spotlight with the rescue of fifteen villagers from the Yamuna during floods. Since then, the rescue saga of choppers has continued. The adage 'Above all, choppers save lives' is apt across the world, and India is no exception. The first VIP sortie was done the same year with Pandit Nehru going to witness an IAF firepower demonstration at Tilpat range near Delhi, because all roads leading to it were jammed!

The smaller Bell 47 III Gs joined the fleet in 1957 for communication, reconnaissance and other difficult 'light duties'. Another first by choppers was an international humanitarian assistance and disaster relief (HADR) deployment, i.e., flood relief in Sri Lanka between December 1957 and January 1958 with two Bells. These helicopters also performed very well during the 1962 war with China, including night sorties in the hills with the help of hand-held torchlights. The first martyr of the fleet, Squadron Leader V.K. Saighal of 105 HU, flew these machines till he was never heard of again after landing at Tsangdhar.

The next magnificent machines brought into the helicopter fleet were Mi-4s inducted from the Soviet Union in November 1957. Their very first gallant acts included extensive flood rescue over the Brahmaputra, support to counter-insurgency forces in then North-East Frontier Agency (NEFA), and support to the police action in Goa in 1961. But the real action came while supporting the Indian Army in 1962. The exemplary support to the army in NEFA, as also the loss of at least three Mi-4s to enemy, fire is well recorded. There were gallant stories from Ladakh too. One of them was aerial support under hostile fire to a besieged garrison at Galwan. Finally, an entire company was whisked away to safety under the very noses of the Chinese. The gallant action of the Indian Army at Walong was fully supported by IAF helicopters, who were hit by Chinese fire many times. Some of the chopper heroes awarded gallantry medals were Badhawar, Narayanan, Williams and Saini.

These workhorses contributed much more in the 1965 war with Pakistan. Innovation and adaptability against a non-conventional operation by Pakistani Razakars threw up great moments. One was the literal overnight modification of the Mi-4s into a bombing and strafing role. Almost eighty offensive missions were carried out, besides more than a thousand logistics support and casualty evacuation sorties. Before this, the Mi-4s of 110 HU had helped to win the Mizo Conflict of 1964, made famous because of the strafing by fighter aircraft of various hotspots of Mizoram.

It was the 1971 war that brought jointness to a peak. Mi-4s, under Eastern Air Command, allowed the impossible to happen under a crazy but brilliant army corps commander. General Sagat Singh utilized Mi-4s carrying fully armed troops to hop across rivers and numerous riverine channels by night to shock and awe two Pakistani brigades. Nowhere in the original plan, General Sagat's troops reached the doors of Dacca, much to the surprise of General Niazi, and even the Indian Army. This cocktail of Gurkhas and Mi-4s proved to be too strong for all and brought in vogue the lexicon of special heli-borne operations in the Indian armed forces. The Mi-4s were finally retired in 1981.

The next workhorses to come in were the Mi-8s in 1972. They were the backbone of support to counter-insurgency forces in the Northeast in the 1980s and 1990s. They virtually did everything and everywhere, including deployment in Sierra Leone as UN peacekeepers. Operation Khukri, where a large garrison of mostly Indian peacekeepers were supported over months and then rescued, calls for a separate book. However, it was the Herculean effort in Sri Lanka in 1986–89 where this fleet truly earned laurels for itself. Every conceivable role in joint operations was executed, and with what elan! Starting off with the infamous heli-borne operations at Jaffna University to millions of tons of supplies at hundreds of helipads to an effective armed role, the Mi-8s did it all.

The beginning of the 1980s saw an upgradation of the fleet at breakneck speed: Mi-25s (attack choppers) in 1984, Mi-26s (the largest chopper) in 1985, and Mi-17s (future workhorses) in 1986. It was an eventful time with the Siachen Glacier battle raging on one side, IPKF on the other, and to top it, Operation Falcon in the Northeast. Today, after the recent imbroglio at Doklam, people forget that a much larger riposte was given to our not-so-friendly neighbour way back in 1986–87.

## Operation Falcon/Chequerboard (1986–87)

On 16 June 1986, Chinese troops intruded into Sumdorong Chu Valley in Arunachal Pradesh and started building permanent structures. This was discovered by 12 Assam Regiment when they returned after the winter withdrawal. Some 200 Chinese soldiers continued to illegally occupy the area despite formal protests by the Government of India. By August, they had constructed a helipad and air supply had started. In response, an entire brigade of 5 Mountain Division was airlifted by the IAF's Mi-8s and the newer, more powerful Mi-17s to Zimithang, which overlooked Sumdorong Chu. In response to massive Chinese mobilization from Chengdu and Lanzhou, the Indian Army and IAF launched Operation Chequerboard to move ten divisions and a number of IAF fighter and helicopter squadrons. Three divisions of the Indian Army, mobilized in the Arunachal sector, were entirely supplied by IAF Mi-17s till mid-1987. This was a record effort from the IAF's helicopter fleet, which is not very well documented or acknowledged.

As I said at the beginning of the book, the stories and incidents in this book are just a snapshot of the IAF's helicopter legacy. This book is every chopper pilot's story—I was just lucky to be in the right place at the right time. In tune with his or her very unstable machine, a chopper pilot is always ready for the uncertain and the unexpected. So don't expect him or her to be laid-back when doing anything else too!

# ABOUT THE AUTHOR

**Air Vice Marshal Rajesh Isser (retd)** is an experienced military aviator with extensive operational and combat experience, including in Sri Lanka (IPKF), at the Siachen Glacier, during the Kargil War and in the Congo (UNPK 2003–04). He has been a task force commander in many rescue and relief operations across India, and been awarded by six Indian states for his work. He has also participated in rescue operations in South Asian and African countries. This is his fourth book.